EasyTerms™
Terminology Guidebook
for Human Anatomy and Physiology

Copyright 2009, Ed Creager

This edition of EasyTerms is one in a series of simple-to-use, college-level terminology guidebooks.

Although these guidebooks were originally intended for college students, many High School students will also find them helpful as they prepare for college.

Other topics to be covered in forthcoming editions:

- Biochemistry
- Biology
- Botany
- Business Management
- Cell Biology
- Ecology
- Genetics
- Microbiology
- Nursing
- Nutrition
- Psychology
- Zoology

EasyTerms can help support your educational advancement and can boost the vocabulary of almost anyone who reads it.

For more information on these and other publications, please visit the author's site:

www.edcreager.blogspot.com

… and please note the author's "signature book" entitled,

"The Money-Saving Idea Book: Inside Tips for Starving Students, Frugal Seniors and Every Financial Survivor."

("The Money-Saving Idea Book" © and TM , Ed Creager, 2009.)

Foreword

This Human Anatomy and Physiology edition is a simple-to-use, college-level* terminology guidebook and is part of the EasyTerms reference series. In the book, terms are arranged alphabetically within appropriate topic areas. The complete index makes it easy to find any term and its definition.

* These books can also help High School students prepare so that, before they attend college, they'll already know a considerable amount of the terminology they'll need.

A substantial number of the terms defined here have additional definitions outside the scope of the subject being covered. More general definitions and additional meanings, if sought, are to be found in less specialized publications such as dictionaries and encyclopedias.

Please check the website of the author...

www.edcreager.blogspot.com

for more information on other available books.

To buy the Biology edition of EasyTerms and receive a **Preferred Customer Discount of 25%**, please go to www.tinyurl.com/bookonbiology, click on "Add to Cart," and enter the **discount code "EQ99TEC8 "** during check-out.

To save 25% on the Nutrition edition, go to www.tinyurl.com/bookonnutrition and after clicking "Add to Cart," enter the **discount code "GBCN9U7M".**

Important Notice:

The resources provided hereby, including websites, books and related materials, are intended to provide accurate information regarding the subject matter. All products and services are provided with the understanding that neither the author nor the publisher is engaged in rendering legal, accounting, or other professional advice. If expert assistance is needed, the services of a competent professional should be obtained.

EasyTerms™
Terminology Guidebook
Table of Contents

The terms that follow are divided into the topics shown below. The page number on which the topic begins is given. Within each topic, the terms are arranged alphabetically.

The Human Body as a Whole

1. abdomen

Body region between the diaphragm and the pelvis.

2. abdominopelvic

Of or in the abdominal and pelvic regions.

3. anatomical position

A standing position with palms of hands turned the same direction as the face.

4. anatomy

The study of structure.

5. anterior

Ventral, toward the belly.

6. appendicular

Of the appendages.

7. axilla

Armpit.

8. biocybernetic

Concerning a living automatic self-controlling system.

9. caudal

Toward the tail, or inferior part of body.

10. cephalic

Of or toward the head; in humans, superior.

11. complementarity

A relationship in which structures and their functions are mutually reinforcing.

12. controlled output

Output of a body process determined by an automatic control system.

13. coronal

Crownlike; of the crown of the head.

14. cranial

Pertaining to the cranium.

15. cybernetic system

A self-controlling, automatic regulatory system.

16. distal

Most distant from the point of origin of a structure.

17. dorsal

Toward the back; posterior in humans.

18. dynamic equilibrium

The maintenance of balance in motion; the preservation of nearly constant internal conditions.

19. epigastric

Of the upper middle portion of the abdomen.

20. excitability

Responsiveness to a stimulus.

21. extrinsic

Originating outside an organism.

22. feedback

The use of the output of a process to influence the process.

23. homeostasis

The maintenance of a narrow, tolerable range of internal conditions.

24. homeostatic system

A control system that regulates internal conditions.

25. hypochondriac

Of the abdominal region inferior to the ribs; having anxiety about health.

26. hypogastric

Of the abdominal region inferior to the stomach.

27. in vitro

In glass; in an artificial environment.

28. in vivo

In the body.

29. inferior

Below or beneath.

30. inguinal

Of the groin.

31. internal

Inside or within.

32. internal environment

The environment around cells, but within the body.

33. interstitial

Concerning spaces between cells.

34. lateral

On or toward the side.

35. lumbar

In the region of the lower back.

36. median

Toward or in the middle.

37. mediastinum

Enclosed cavity between the lungs that contains the heart, trachea, and part of the esophagus.

38. negative feedback

A control system in which a system's output inhibits activity of the system.

39. operating set point

Hypothetical average value around which a condition is maintained.

40. organ

A structure made up of several tissues that carries out particular functions; component of a system.

41. organ system

Body system comprised of several organs that work together.

42. organizational complexity

A concept that concerns the structural levels of an organism.

43. oscillation

Continuous variation of a condition over the same range.

44. pectoral

Of the chest.

45. peripheral

Outer or away from the center.

46. peritonitis

Inflammation of the peritoneum, or lining of the abdominal cavity.

47. physiology

The study of life functions.

48. positive feedback

Output from a system that accelerates change in the system.

49. posterior

Toward the rear, dorsal in humans.

50. process

An outgrowth or protrusion; an ongoing action.

51. prone

Lying horizontally and face down.

52. proximal

Nearest the point of origin of a structure.

53. reflex

An automatic involuntary response to a stimulus.

54. sagittal

A plane dividing right and left sides.

55. section

Plane through the body or an organ.

56. sensor

A devise that detects a stimulus, often as a component of a control system.

57. serous fluid

Watery secretion from a serous membrane.

58. signal

That which conveys information.

59. stimulus

A change in the environment detectable by a receptor.

60. superficial

On or near the body surface.

61. superior

Of the head or upper body regions.

62. supine

Lying horizontally with face up.

63. systemic

Concerning the whole body.

64. thoracic

Of the chest.

65. thorax

Chest; body region above diaphragm.

66. tissue

A group of similar cells, including intercellular substances, that carry out a particular function.

67. transverse

Crosswise.

68. umbilical

Of the umbilicus.

69. umbilicus

Site where umbilical cord was attached to fetus; navel.

70. ventral

Of or toward the belly.

71. viscera

Internal organs.

72. visceral

Of the viscera.

The Chemical Level of Function

73. acid

An ionizing substance that donates hydrogen ions.

74. adenosine triphosphate

An important energy storage molecule.

75. alkaline

Basic, able to accept hydrogen ions.

76. amino acid

A molecule having both acid and amino functional groups.

77. anion

A negatively charge ion.

78. atom

Smallest particle that retains properties of an element.

79. atomic number

The number of protons in the nucleus of an atom.

80. atomic symbol

One- or two-letter code used to stand for a particular element.

81. atomic weight

The total number of protons and neutrons in an atom; the average number if there are isotopes of the element.

82. base

An ionizing substance that accepts hydrogen ions or reacts with an acid to form a salt.

83. bioenergetics

The science of energy changes in living systems.

84. buffer

A substance that resists pH change by holding or releasing hydrogen ions in a solution.

85. carbohydrate

An organic compound having several alcohol groups and an aldehyde or ketone group.

86. catalyst

A substance that increases a chemical reaction rate.

87. cation

A positively charged ion.

88. cellulose

Fibrous carbohydrate that forms the structure of many plants and provides insoluble fiber in the human diet.

89. chemical bond

Any force produced by interacting electrons that helps to hold molecules together.

90. chemical energy

Energy stored in molecules.

91. cholesterol

Animal steroid found in cell membranes.

92. coenzyme

Simple, nonprotein substance that works with an enzyme.

93. colloid

Glue-like; a particle in a colloidal dispersion.

94. colloidal dispersion

A state of matter with small particles suspended in a medium.

95. compound

A substance with two or more elements combined in definite proportion.

96. covalent bond

A chemical bond formed by shared electrons between two atoms.

97. dehydration

Removal of water.

98. denaturation

An alteration in the shape and properties of a protein molecule.

99. deoxyribonuclease

An enzyme that digests DNA.

100. deoxyribonucleic acid (DNA)

A nucleic acid in chromosomes that directs protein synthesis and transmits genetic information to a new generation.

101. disaccharide

A molecule having two sugar (saccharide) units held together by a glycosidic bond.

102. electron

A negatively charged particle that continually moves around the nucleus of an atom.

103. element

A fundamental unit of matter.

104. endergonic

Requiring energy, as in a chemical reaction.

105. entropy

Tendency toward chaos or disorder.

106. enzyme

A protein that increases the rate of a chemical reaction in a living organism.

107. exergonic

Releasing energy, as in a chemical reaction.

108. fatty acid

A long hydrocarbon chain with a carboxyl group at one end.

109. functional group

A component of a molecule that participates in a chemical reaction.

110. glucose

Main blood sugar.

111. glycerol

Alcohol to which fatty acids are bound in fats.

112. glycine

An amino acid with the simplest chemical structure.

113. glycolipid

A molecule that contains both carbohydrate and lipid components.

114. glycoprotein

A molecule that contains both carbohydrate and protein components.

115. gram molecular weight

The quantity of a substance (in grams) equal to its molecular weight.

116. hydrogen bond

Weak covalent bond between hydrogen and another element, such as oxygen or nitrogen.

117. hydrolysis

The splitting of a molecule with the addition of water.

118. hydrophilic

Attacted to water.

119. hydrophobic

Tending to avoid water.

120. ion

A charged atom or group of atoms.

121. ionic bond

A chemical bond with atoms held together by the attraction of unlike charges.

122. **isomer**

A molecule having the same kinds and number of atoms as another molecule, but arranged differently.

123. **isotope**

An atom having a different number of neutrons than certain other atoms of the same element.

124. **kinetic**

Energy of motion.

125. **lactic acid**

Product of anaerobic metabolism especially in skeletal muscle.

126. **lecithin**

A phospholipid characteristic of animal tissues.

127. **lipid**

Any fat or fatlike substance.

128. **mixture**

Two or more substances combined in any proportions and retaining their individual properties.

129. **mole**

A gram molecular weight.

130. **molecule**

The smallest quantity of a substance that retains its chemical properties.

131. **monosaccharide**

A simple sugar.

132. neutron

An uncharged particle in the nucleus of an atom.

133. nonpolar

Uncharged; lacking polarity.

134. nucleic acid

A polymer of nucleotides; DNA or RNA.

135. nucleotide

A molecule having a nitrogenous base, a 5-carbon sugar, and one or more phosphates.

136. nucleus

Central part of an atom or a cell; a group of cell bodies in the central nervous system.

137. organic

Containing carbon.

138. oxidation

Addition of oxygen or loss of electrons in a chemical reaction.

139. peptide bond

A chemical bond between the amino group of one amino acid and the carboxyl group of another.

140. pH

A scale for expressing acidity or alkalinity; the negative logarithm of the hydrogen ion concentration.

141. phospholipid

A lipid made of glycerol, fatty acids, and phosphoric acid.

142. polar compound

A molecule having a charged area or polarity.

143. polymer

A molecule consisting of repeating units.

144. polypeptide

A chain of amino acids held together by peptide bonds.

145. polysaccharide

A molecule consisting of many saccharide units connected by glycosidic bonds.

146. potential energy

Energy due to position and capable of being released, as in a rock at the top of a hill.

147. protein

A polymer of amino acids.

148. proton

A positively charged particle in the nucleus of an atom.

149. radiation

Spreading from a center; giving off electromagnetic particles and waves.

150. radioactivity

Spontaneous decay of an isotope with emission of particles and energy.

151. radioisotope

Isotope that displays radioactivity.

152. reactant

A substance that is changed by a chemical reaction.

153. reduction

Gain of an electron or loss of oxygen in a chemical reaction.

154. ribonucleic acid (RNA)

A nucleic acid made from information in DNA that is involved in protein synthesis.

155. salt

Compound that fully ionizes in solution.

156. saturated fatty acid

A fatty acid lacking double bonds in the carbon chain and being saturated with hydrogen.

157. saturation

Condition of having all chemical affinities satisfied.

158. specific heat

The amount of heat needed to increase the temperature of a specific volume of substance one degree Celsius.

159. specificity

The attribute of being specific.

160. stereoisomer

Compound having the same kind and number of atoms as another compound, but in a different spatial arrangement.

161. steroid

A lipid with a complex four-ring structure.

162. suspension

Dispersal of particles in a liquid.

163. template

Pattern.

164. trace element

A chemical element normally present in very small amounts in the body.

165. triglyceride

A triacylglycerol (glycerol and three fatty acids).

166. unsaturated fatty acid

Fatty acid with pairs of hydrogen atoms replaced by double bonds in the carbon chain.

167. uridine triphosphate (UTP)

A high energy molecule.

168. valence

An ion's charge.

The Cellular Level of Function

169. active transport

Transport of a substance against a gradient using a carrier molecule, enzyme, and cellular energy.

170. adsorptive endocytosis

Entry of a substance into a cell by first attaching to the cell membrane.

171. anaphase

A mitotic stage during which chromosomes move apart.

172. anticodon

A three-base sequence of transfer RNA that fits with a particular codon on messenger RNA.

173. benign

Nonmalignant, favorable for recovery.

174. binding site

A site where a particular molecule binds to a membrane or other structure.

175. bulk flow

Streaming of molecules that allows them to move faster than by diffusion.

176. cachexia

Wasting, weakness, and weight-loss seen especially in cancer patients.

177. cancer

Malignant, invasive tumor that grows by uncontrolled cell division.

178. carcinogen

A cancer-inducing agent.

179. carrier

A transfer molecule; a person capable of transmitting an unexpressed gene.

180. carrier saturation

A condition with all carrier molecules carrying a substance.

181. cell

A basic functional unit of a living organism.

182. cell cycle

A repetitive sequence of events in DNA replication and cell division.

183. cell membrane

Lipid and protein compounds that form the boundary of a cell.

184. cell theory

A theory stating that living things are composed of cells.

185. centriole

One of a pair of intracellular bodies that participate in forming a mitotic spindle.

186. chromatin

Nuclear material that condenses into distinct chromosomes during cell division.

187. chromosome

In a human cell, one of 46 nuclear structures made of DNA and protein.

188. chrononcology

The use of cell division rhythms to schedule cancer therapy.

189. chronotherapy

The use of any rhythms to schedule therapy.

190. cilium

A tiny hairlike projection found on some epithelial cells.

191. cisterna

Reservoir or cavity.

192. codon

A three-base sequence in messenger RNA derived from DNA and specifying amino acid placement in a protein.

193. colloidal osmotic pressure

Pressure exerted on a membrane by colloidal particles, such as blood proteins.

194. complementary base pairing

Bonding between certain bases in nucleic acid strands.

195. concentration gradient

Range of concentrations of a substance from one region to another.

196. cytokinesis

Division of the cytoplasm that follows division of a nucleus.

197. cytoplasm

Cell substance, excluding the nucleus.

198. cytoskeleton

The organelles forming a cell's internal framework.

199. cytosol

The fluid part of cytoplasm that suspends organelles.

200. deletion

Loss of one or more bases from a DNA strand.

201. DNA polymerase

An enzyme that increases chain length in DNA synthesis.

202. DNA replication

Synthesis of new DNA according to information in an existing DNA template.

203. endocytosis

Movement of particles across a membrane into a cell.

204. endoplasmic reticulum

A membranous vesicular network within a cell.

205. exocytosis

The movement of particles across a membrane out of a cell.

206. extracellular

Outside a cell.

207. facilitated diffusion

Diffusion down a gradient on a carrier molecule but not requiring cellular energy.

208. filtration

Passage of a fluid across a membrane by mechanical pressure.

209. flagellum

A movable hairlike process on a cell.

210. fluid-mosaic model

A model of molecular arrangements in a cell membrane.

211. frameshift mutation

A DNA sequence change caused by adding or deleting bases.

212. gel

The semi-solid state of a colloidal dispersion.

213. genetic code

The three-base sequences in messenger RNA derived from a DNA template that determine amino acid order in proteins.

214. Golgi apparatus

Membranous vesicles clustered in cells that complete synthesis of secretions.

215. gradient

The rate of change in the magnitude of concentration, pressure, or other variable.

216. haploid

Having one of a pair of chromosomes.

217. hydrostatic pressure

Force exerted by a fluid.

218. hyperosmotic

Having higher osmotic pressure than a reference solution.

219. hypertonic

Causing movement of water out of cells.

220. hyposmotic

Having lower osmotic pressure than a reference solution.

221. hypotonic

Causing movement of water into cells.

222. integral

Relating to an inseparable component.

223. interphase

A cell cycle stage during which the cell is not dividing.

224. intracellular

Within a cell.

225. intrinsic

Entirely within.

226. isosmotic

Having the same osmotic pressure as a reference solution.

227. isotonic

Causing no net water movement across a cell membrane.

228. isozyme

An isomer of an enzyme; one of two or more forms of an enzyme that catalyze the same reaction.

229. ligand

That which binds to a receptor.

230. lysosome

Membrane-bound organelle that contains digestive enzymes.

231. malignancy

A tendency to become more virulent; a cancerous growth.

232. malignant

Cancerous; tending to become more virulent.

233. messenger RNA (mRNA)

A nucleic acid that carries information as codons for protein synthesis.

234. metaphase

A mitotic stage during which chromosomes align along the equator of a cell.

235. metastasis

The transfer of disease from one organ to another.

236. microfilament

A small, hollow protein fiber in cytoplasm that aids in movement or forms part of a cytoskeleton.

237. microtubule

A cylindrical organelle that forms part of a cell's mitotic spindle.

238. mitochondrion

An organelle that contains enzymes for oxidative and energy-capturing processes.

239. mitosis

Nuclear division that produces two identical nuclei.

240. mutagen

An agent that can alter DNA.

241. nuclear

Of the nucleus.

242. nucleolus

A body containing RNA within a nucleus.

243. nucleoplasm

The substance of a nucleus.

244. organelle

A functional unit inside a cell.

245. osmolarity

A solution's osmotic concentration determined by the number of osmotically active particles it contains.

246. osmosis

Diffusion of water from its own region of higher water concentration to a region of lower water concentration.

247. osmotic pressure

Pressure created by osmosis.

248. passive transport

A process that moves substances without energy expenditure by the organism.

249. permeability

Membrane property that allows molecules and ions to pass through.

250. peroxisome

An organelle that contains catalase and other oxidative enzymes.

251. phagocytosis

Engulfment into a vacuole and digestion by a scavenger cell.

252. pinocytosis

Intake of extracellular fluid by cells; cell drinking.

253. plasma membrane

Membrane forming the boundary of a cell.

254. prophase

The first mitotic stage during which the chromosomes become distinct.

255. protoplasm

Cell substance; literally, first formed.

256. receptor

A specific site where a particular substance can bind.

257. remission

Abatement of disease symptoms or the period during which the abatement occurs.

258. replication

Duplication.

259. ribosomal RNA (rRNA)

A nucleic acid that forms part of a ribosome.

260. ribosome

An organelle containing ribonucleic acid and protein where protein synthesis occurs.

261. secretion

A cell product; the act of transporting a substance across a membrane.

262. selectively permeable

A membrane property that allows passage of some substances while preventing passage of others.

263. sodium-potassium pump

Mechanism that actively moves Na ions out of cells and K ions into them against gradients.

264. sol

A liquid state of a colloidal dispersion.

265. solute

A dissolved substance.

266. solution

A liquid containing dissolved substances.

267. solvent

A substance in which other substances can dissolve.

268. surface tension

Resistance to rupture by the surface film of a liquid.

269. surface-to-volume ratio

The surface area of a structure divided by its volume.

270. telophase

The last mitotic stage during which nuclei reform.

271. teratogen

An agent that causes defective embryonic development.

272. tonicity

The degree to which fluid can move into or out of cells.

273. transcription

The transfer of coded genetic information from DNA to mRNA.

274. transfer RNA (tRNA)

RNA that carries amino acids to specific sites in a growing peptide chain.

275. translation

The process by which mRNA codons are used to determine the sequence of amino acids in a protein.

276. triacylglycerol

A lipid molecule containing glycerol and three fatty acids.

277. tubulin

A protein that forms intracellular microtubules.

278. tumor

Abnormal aggregation of cells that can be malignant or benign.

279. tumor necrosis factor

A substance that causes degeneration and death of tumor cells.

280. vesicle

A small sac filled with liquid.

The Tissue Level of Function

281. abscess

Localized accumulation of pus and necrotic tissue.

282. acinus

A small cluster.

283. adipose

Pertaining to fat.

284. apocrine

A gland thought to lose part of its substance with its secretions.

285. blastocyst

Hollow ball of cells that arises early in embryonic development.

286. bradykinin

A polypeptide with a potent vasodilating action.

287. cardiac muscle

Muscle tissue found in the heart, characterized by the presence of intercalated disks.

288. cartilage

A firm, resilient, flexible connective tissue.

289. cartilaginous

Consisting of cartilage.

290. chondroblast

A cell that lays down matrix in cartilage.

291. chondrocyte

A mature cartilage cell.

292. collagen

A fibrous protein in connective tissue.

293. connective tissue

Tissue in which fibrocytes make fibers and ground substance.

294. cryostat

A device that maintains a low temperature.

295. cuboidal

Cube-shaped.

296. desmosome

A structure that holds cells together along adjacent membranes.

297. differentiation

The specialization of structures during embyronic development.

298. ectoderm

The outermost germ layer in an embryo.

299. elastin

Main protein in elastic fibers of connective tissues.

300. endoderm

The innermost germ layer in an embryo.

301. epithelial

Of epithelium.

302. epithelium

A thin tissue that lines hollow organs or covers surfaces.

303. exocrine

Of a gland with ducts.

304. exudate

Fluid, pus, or cells deposited in a tissue or on a body surface.

305. fibroblast

A connective tissue cell that makes fibers and ground substance.

306. fibrocyte

Mature fibroblast that maintains fibrous matrix of a connective tissue.

307. gap junction

Connection between two adjacent cells formed by transmembrane proteins called connexons.

308. goblet cell

Single-celled gland that produces mucus.

309. ground substance

A glycoprotein deposited among fibers of connective tissue.

310. Haversian system

A set of concentric lamellae around a canal in compact bone.

311. histiocyte

A tissue macrophage.

312. histologist

A scientist who studies tissues.

313. histology

The study of tissues.

314. holocrine

A gland that secretes whole cells and their products.

315. intercalated

Inserted between other structures.

316. intercellular

Between cells.

317. intercellular matrix

Material deposited between cells, such as in connective tissues.

318. lacuna

Cavity.

319. lamella

Layer (usually one of several).

320. **lamina**

Thin, flat plate.

321. **matrix**

A fibrous framework in which ground substance of connective tissue is deposited.

322. **merocrine**

A gland that secretes its product by exocytosis.

323. **mesoderm**

The middle germ layer in an embryo.

324. **morula**

A solid ball of cells in early embryological development.

325. **mucin**

A glycoprotein in ground substance and mucous secretions.

326. **mucous**

Pertaining to mucus.

327. **mucous membrane**

Membrane that contains goblet cells that secrete mucus.

328. **mucus**

Thick secretion from a goblet cell.

329. **necrosis**

Tissue death from injury or disease.

330. neuron

Cell of the nervous system that conducts impulses, and secretes and responds to neurotransmitters.

331. osteoblast

A cell that forms fibers and ground substance of bone.

332. osteoclast

A cell that digests bone matrix.

333. osteocyte

A mature bone cell occupying a lacuna.

334. perichondrium

A connective tissue membrane covering cartilage.

335. phagocyte

Cell that can engulf and destroy debris, foreign particles, and other cells.

336. pseudostratified

Appearing to have layers that are not actually present.

337. pus

A product of inflammation consisting of debris from dead leukocytes and microorganisms.

338. reticular

Of a net or meshwork.

339. scab

A crust over a superficial wound.

340. scar

Connective tissue that has replaced an injured tissue unable to replace itself.

341. skeletal muscle

Muscle attached to bones, characterized by striations and absence of intercalated disks.

342. stratum

A layer, usually of tissue.

343. tight junction

Region of fused membranes of adjacent cells.

The Integumentary System

344. arrector pili

Small muscles associated with hair follicles that can cause hairs to stand upright.

345. cutaneous

Of the skin.

346. cuticle

The outer layer of skin, especially around nails.

347. dermal papilla

An extension of dermis into the epidermis.

348. dermis

A thick skin layer underlying the epidermis.

349. eccrine

Excretory.

350. eleidin

A keratin precursor found in the stratum lucidum.

351. endochondral

Within cartilage.

352. epidermis

Outer skin layer consisting of epithelium.

353. eponychium

Skin fold over a nail root.

354. hair follicle

Connective tissue sheath containing epithelial cells from which a hair develops.

355. hypodermis

Tissue beneath the skin.

356. hyponychium

Cornified epithelium under a free nail border.

357. integumentary

Of the skin.

358. keratin

Water-insoluble protein in skin, hair, and nails.

359. keratinocyte

A skin cell that contains keratin.

360. keratohyalin

A translucent substance in skin.

361. lanugo

Fine hair on the skin of a fetus.

362. lunula

Whitish crescent at nail base; literally, half moon.

363. melanin

A dark brown pigment of hair and skin.

364. melanocyte

A cell that makes melanin.

365. melanoma

A common kind of skin cancer.

366. papilla

A nipple-shaped projection.

367. piloerection

The standing on end of hairs.

368. pilus

A hair.

369. sebaceous

Of sebum.

370. sebum

A substance containing oils and epithelial cell debris from sebaceous glands.

371. subcutaneous

Beneath the skin.

372. sudoriferous

Secreting sweat.

373.   sudoriferous gland

Sweat gland.

Bone Tissues and Bones

374. bone remodeling

Continuous deposition and reabsorption of bone in response to mechanical and chemical factors.

375. calcification

Depositing of calcium salts in an organic matrix.

376. callus

A thickened area.

377. canaliculus

A tiny canal.

378. cancellous

Spongy.

379. closed reduction

Nonsurgical bone realignment after a fracture.

380. comminuted

Broken into small pieces, as in a splintered bone.

381. condyle

A large rounded protrusion at a bone end.

382. condyloid

Like a condyle.

383. coronoid

A sharp process on a bone; resembling a crow's beak.

384. endosteum

Membranous lining of a marrow cavity.

385. epicondyle

A bone protrusion to which a muscle attaches.

386. epiphyseal

Pertaining to the epiphysis of a bone or the growth region near it.

387. facet

Smooth, flat articular surface on a bone.

388. fissure

A furrow of slit.

389. foramen

Opening or hole.

390. fossa

A depression in the surface of a bone.

391. fracture

A break, such as in a bone.

392. hydroxyapatite

A mineral that makes up the bulk of bone.

393. intramembranous

Within a membrane.

394. ligament

Cord of fibrous connective tissue that attaches bones to each other.

395. marrow

Fatty substance found in a marrow cavity.

396. meatus

External opening of a canal.

397. medullary

Pertaining to the inner part or core of an organ.

398. mesenchyme

Embryonic mesoderm.

399. open reduction

Surgical repair of a fractured bone.

400. ossification

Mineral deposition in the process of bone formation.

401. osteogenesis

The development of bone.

402. osteoid

Resembling bone.

403. osteomalacia

Adult bone softening as a result of a vitamin deficiency.

404. osteon

The cells, matrix, and passages that make up a unit of compact bone.

405. osteoporosis

Abnormal porousness of bone, which makes it fracture-prone.

406. periosteum

A membranous covering on the surface of a bone.

407. raphe

A seamlike ridge, usually where two structures have fused.

408. rickets

A failure of bones to harden in childhood because of a calcium deficiency.

409. sesamoid

Referring to a bone formed in a tendon; like a sesame seed.

410. sinus

A cavity or recess.

411. spicule

A needle-shaped structure.

412. sulcus

A furrow or groove.

413. sutural

Of a suture.

414. suture

A fibrous joint at which no movement occurs.

415. trabecula

A rod-like structure; a spicule of spongy bone.

416. trochanter

A large, rounded process on a bone.

417. tubercle

A small, rounded protrusion on a bone.

418. tuberosity

A protrusion from a bone surface to which muscles attach.

419. Volkmann's canal

Channel for blood vessels and nerves through the matrix of bone to Haversian systems.

420. Wormian bone

A small accessory bone that can form between larger skull bones.

421. xiphoid

A swordshaped process of the sternum.

422. zygomatic

Of the cheek bone.

The Skeleton

423. acetabulum

Cup-shaped depression in lateral surface of os coxa into which the head of the femur fits.

424. atlas

First cervical vertebra, which articulates with the occipital bone of the skull.

425. axial

Referring to the body's axis.

426. axis

Second cervical vertebra, which has a projection (dens) around which the atlas rotates.

427. calcaneus

Heelbone.

428. carpal

A wrist bone.

429. centrum

An anatomical center.

430. cervical

Of a neck.

431. clavicle

Bone that extends from the sternum to the scapula.

432. coccygeal

Referring to the coccyx.

433. coccyx

The caudal end of the spinal column; tail bone.

434. concha

One of several shell-shaped bones in the nasal cavity.

435. contraction

Developing tension or shortening, as in a muscle fiber.

436. costal

Of a rib.

437. coxal bone

A bone that forms half of the pelvic girdle.

438. cranium

Skull bones that surround the brain.

439. cribriform

Sieve-like.

440. crista

Crest or ridge.

441. cuneate

Triangular.

442. cuneiform

Wedge-shaped.

443. diaphysis

The long slender part of a long bone.

444. diploe

Loose boony tissue between two outer plates, as in some cranial bones.

445. epiphysis

The end region of a long bone.

446. ethmoid

Sieve-like.

447. fibula

Lateral leg bone found between the knee and ankle.

448. fontanel

A membranous non-bony region between cranial bones in an infant.

449. frontal

Of the forehead.

450. gladiolus

A sword-shaped part of the sternum.

451. humerus

The bone of the upper arm.

452. iliac

Of the ilium.

453. ilium

The posteriolateral bone of the pelvis.

454. incus

Anvil; the ear bone that receives vibrations from the malleus.

455. interosseous

Lying in between bones.

456. ischium

A posterior bone of the pelvic girdle.

457. lambdoidal

Ridge-like suture of the skull; literally like the Greek letter lambda.

458. malleus

Hammer; the outermost bone of the middle ear.

459. mandibular

Of the mandible.

460. manubrium

Handle; the part of the sternum that articulates with the clavicles.

461. mastoid

Nipple-like; region the temporal bone behind the ear.

462. maxilla

The upper bone bone that contains sockets for upper teeth.

463. maxillary

Of the maxilla.

464. metacarpal

One of five bones in the palm of the hand.

465. metatarsal

One of five long bones in the foot.

466. nucleus pulposus

A jellylike substance found inside an intervertebral disc.

467. occipital

Of or near the back of the head.

468. ossicle

Middle ear bone.

469. osteoarthritis

A chronic inflammatory, degenerative joint disease.

470. palatine

Of the palate.

471. parietal

Of the wall of a cavity.

472. patella

A small bone that forms the kneecap.

473. pectoral girdle

Clavicles and scapulas, bones that attach arms to axial skeleton.

474. pedicle

A bony process between the lamina and centrum of a vertebra.

475. pelvic

Of the pelvis.

476. pelvic girdle

Coxal bones that attach legs to axial skeleton.

477. pelvis

Basin-like bony lower portion of trunk.

478. petrous

Rock-like.

479. phalanges

Small, slightly elongated bones of the fingers and toes.

480. pubis

An anterior bone of the pelvic girdle.

481. pubofemoral

Of the pubic and femoral regions.

482. radial

Of the radius.

483. radius

The smaller of the forearm bones.

484. sacral

Of the sacrum.

485. sacrum

A bone formed from the fusion of five vertebrae that articulates posteriorly with the pelvic girdle.

486. scapula

A large bone lateral to the vertebrae in the shoulder area.

487. sclerotome

An embryonic tissue that gives rise to vertebrae and ribs.

488. sella turcica

A saddle-shaped depression in the sphenoid bone in which the pituitary gland is located; literally, Turkish saddle.

489. sphenoid

Winglike; a skull bone with winglike processes.

490. spinal

Of the vertebral column.

491. squamous

Scalelike.

492. stapes

The middle ear bone that transmits vibrations to the oval window.

493. styloid

Like a stylus; long thin process on a bone.

494. supraorbital

Above an orbit, such as that of the eye.

495. talus

An ankle bone.

496. tarsal

Of the foot bones.

497. temporal

Time-related; a brain lobe where auditory and olfactory areas are located.

498. tibia

Larger, more medial weight-bearing bone of the leg.

499. transverse process

One of paired projections extending laterally from the neural arch of a vertebra.

500. trochlea

Pulley.

501. ulna

Larger of the forearm bones.

502. vertebral column

Spinal column composed of individual vertebrae and fused vertebrae in the sacrum and coccyx.

503. vomer

A shovel-shaped bone that forms the nasal septum.

Articulations (Joints)

504. abduction

Motion of a body part away from the midline.

505. acromioclavicular

Of the acromion process of the scapula and the clavicle.

506. adduction

Motion toward the body's midline.

507. amphiarthrosis

An immovable or slightly movable joint with articular surfaces connected by cartilage.

508. arthritis

Joint inflammation.

509. arthrosis

A joint.

510. articular

Related to a joint.

511. articular capsule

Two-layered capsule that encloses and protects the joint cavity of a synovial joint.

512. articulation

A joint.

513. atlantoaxial

Of the atlas and axis, the two superiormost vertebrae.

514. atlantooccipital

Of the uppermost vertebra and occipital region of the skull.

515. ball-and-socket joint

A joint with a ball-shaped articular surface of one bone fitting into a socket-shaped articular surface of another.

516. bursa

A sac containing synovial fluid located at pressure points or near joints.

517. bursitis

Inflammation of a bursa.

518. circumduction

Circular motion.

519. contracture

Permanent shortening of a muscle usually associated with injury or disease.

520. coracohumeral

Of the coracoid process of the scapula and the humerus.

521. cruciate

Cross-shaped.

522. diarthrosis

A joint that is freely movable.

523. dislocation

Abnormal displacement of a body part, especially a bone.

524. dorsiflexion

Motion of the toes and foot toward the shin at the ankle joint.

525. elevation

A motion that raises a body part.

526. ellipsoid joint

A joint with oval-shaped articular surfaces.

527. eversion

Turning outward.

528. extension

Motion that increases the angle between two bones.

529. flexion

Motion that decreases the angle between two bones.

530. glenohumeral

Of the glenoid fossa and humerus.

531. glenoid

Socketlike.

532. gliding joint

A joint with articular surfaces that glide over one another.

533. gomphosis

A joint in which a pointed bone fits into a socket, such as a tooth and its socket.

534. hinge joint

A joint with the articulating surfaces moving relative to each other like the parts of a hinge.

535. hyperextension

Extension at a joint beyond the normal range of movement.

536. intervertebral disk

Small flat piece of cartilage between two vertebrae.

537. inversion

Turning inward; a rearrangement in the nucleotide sequence in the DNA of a chromosome.

538. joint

A connection between two or more bones.

539. plantar

Of the sole of the foot.

540. plantarflexion

Motion of the foot and toes downward away from the shin.

541. pronation

Forearm rotation, causing the palm of hand to face backward; placing abdomen downward, as lying in a prone position.

542. protraction

Motion of the mandible forward.

543. retraction

Backward motion, as exemplified by the mandible.

544. rheumatoid arthritis

An autoimmune inflammatory disease affecting joints and other tissues.

545. rotation

Motion of a part about its own axis.

546. sacroiliac

Of the sacrum and ilium.

547. saddle joint

A joint with saddle-shaped articulating surfaces.

548. sprain

An injury in which surrounding tissue is damaged without joint dislocation.

549. sternoclavicular

Of the sternum and clavicle.

550. strain

Stretching of tissues around a joint.

551. supination

Forearm rotation so that the palm of the hand is forward in anatomical position.

552. symphysis

A cartilaginous, slightly moveable joint.

553. synarthrosis

A joint with no intervening tissue between the bones and no movement.

554. synchrondrosis

A slightly moveable or immovable joint with bones connected by cartilage.

555. syndesmosis

A joint with bones bound together by fibrous connective tissue.

556. synostosis

A joint with bones themselves joined by bony material, such as ossified cartilage.

557. synovial

Of a freely movable joint.

558. synovial fluid

Fluid secreted by a synovial membrane into a joint cavity where it lubricates surfaces and nourishes cartilage.

559. synovial joint

Freely movable joint with a joint cavity; diarthrosis.

560. temporomandibular

Of the temporal bone and mandible.

561. tendon

A fibrous connective tissue cord that holds a muscle to a bone.

562. tendon sheath

A synovial membrane around certain tendons, especially at stress points.

Physiology of Muscle Tissue

563. actin

A contractile protein.

564. aerobic

With oxygen.

565. anaerobic

Lacking oxygen.

566. atrophy

A decrease in size, usually accompanied with reduced function.

567. clonus

Rigidity alternating with relaxation in a spasm.

568. contractile protein

A protein that acts in shortening a muscle or causing it to develop tension.

569. contractility

The ability to develop tension or shorten.

570. contraction cycle

Repetitive sliding actions of actin and myosin in a muscle filament as it develops tension.

571. cramp

A spasmodic, painful muscle contraction.

572. creatine phosphate

A molecule that accounts for limited energy storage in muscle.

573. creatinine

A metaboic product of creatine excreted at a constant rate in urine.

574. cross-bridge

The specialized end of a myosin filament that binds to actin during muscle contraction.

575. denervation atrophy

Muscle wasting because of lack of nerve stimulation.

576. disuse atrophy

Muscle wasting because of lack of use.

577. end plate potential

The potential difference at the interface of a muscle fiber and a neuron.

578. epimysium

Connective tissue covering an entire muscle.

579. extensibility

Ability to be extended or stretched.

580. fatigue

Loss of power for a short time.

581. hypertrophy

Increase in the total size of an organ, usually by an increase in the size of its cells.

582. inotropic

Relating to muscle fibers.

583. isometric

Having the same length.

584. latent period

In muscle physiology, a time between the application of a stimulus and the beginning of muscle contraction.

585. motor end plate

A portion of sarcolemma lying beneath nerve endings.

586. motor unit

A motor neuron and the muscle fibers it innervates.

587. muscle fiber

Muscle cell.

588. muscular dystrophy

A disease in which muscles progressively degenerate.

589. myasthenia gravis

Progressive muscle weakening because of an autoimmune reaction at motor end plates.

590. myofibril

A contractile fiber in a muscle cell.

591. myofilament

A component of a myofibril consisting of one or more protein molecules.

592. myogenic

Able to contract automatically without nerve stimulation.

593. myoglobin

A pigmented protein that binds oxygen in muscle tissue.

594. myokinase

An enzyme that makes ATP and AMP from 2 molecules of ADP in muscle tissue.

595. myoneural junction

The structure at which nerve and muscle tissues meet and impulses are relayed.

596. myosin

A protein that comprises thick filaments of a myofibril.

597. myotome

A block of mesoderm from which muscle arises.

598. neuromuscular

Concerning the association between the nervous and muscular systems.

599. oxygen debt

The quantity of oxygen required to oxidize metabolites produced anaerobically during strenuous activity.

600. phosphocreatine

An energy storage molecule found in muscle.

601. plasticity

Able to be molded or formed; changeable.

602. recruitment

A gradual increase in contraction intensity by activation of additional motor units.

603. red muscle

Skeletal muscle having relatively large amounts of myoglobin.

604. rigor mortis

Muscle rigidity of stiffening following death.

605. sarcolemma

The membrane of a muscle cell.

606. sarcomere

The contractile unit of skeletal muscle.

607. sarcoplasm

The protoplasmic, nonfibrillar substance of a muscle cell.

608. sarcoplasmic reticulum

A vesicular network associated with myofibrils of a striated muscle cell.

609. sliding filament theory

An explanation of how myofilaments move with respect to each other during muscle contraction.

610. smooth muscle

A type of muscle located in the walls of hollow organs and blood vessels.

611. spasm

A sudden, violent, involuntary muscle contraction.

612. striation

Stripe.

613. summation

Addition, as in effects of multiple stimuli to a muscle.

614. syncytium

A group of cells that have lost membranes that formerly separated them.

615. tension

A pulling force.

616. tetanus

A sustained contraction maintained by repeated muscle stimulation.

617. tonus

A slight continuous muscle contraction.

618. transverse (T) tubule

Crosswise tubule in skeletal muscle myofibrils that carries signals from the sarcolemma to the myofibrils.

619. treppe

A gradual increase in the strength of muscular contraction following rapidly repeated stimulation.

620. tropomyosin

A muscle protein that alters the actin configuration so that contraction can occur.

621. troponin

A muscle protein that binds to tropomyosin causing it to alter the configuration of actin.

622. **twitch**

A muscle response to a single stimulus.

623. **white muscle**

Muscle that contain relatively little myoglobin.

Muscle Actions

624. Achilles tendon

A tendon in the heel.

625. action

A movement produced by one or more muscles.

626. agonist

The prime mover among a group of muscles.

627. antagonist

A muscle that opposes an angonist.

628. aponeurosis

A fibrous connective tissue sheet to which muscles attach.

629. biceps

Two-headed muscle.

630. deltoid

A large, triangular muscle covering the shoulder joint; like the Greek letter delta.

631. diaphragm

A thin partition, as is formed by a muscle between the thoracic and abdominal cavities.

632. effector

Muscle, gland, or other organ that can be activated by a nerve impulse.

633. endomysium

Connective tissue that covers individual muscle fibers.

634. excitation-contraction coupling

The means by which neural signals excite muscle cells and cause contraction.

635. fascia

Fibrous connective tissue sheath around muscles and beneath skin.

636. fascicle

Bundle, as of muscle fibers.

637. fasciculation

Involuntary twitching of a muscle fiber bundle.

638. fasciculus

A small bundle of fibers.

639. fixator

Muscle that immobilizes one or several bones.

640. fulcrum

Fixed point about which a lever produces movement.

641. gracile

Delicate and slender.

642. insertion

The most moveable attachment of a muscle to a bone.

643. involuntary

Responding to internal signals and not under conscious control.

644. linea alba

Connective tissue at the midline of the anterior abdominal wall; literally, white line.

645. origin

The least movable attachment of a muscle to a bone.

646. perimysium

A connective tissue sheath around a bundle of skeletal muscle fibers.

647. prime mover

A muscle that is the most direct cause of a particular movement.

648. prolapse

A falling or sinking from a normal position.

649. rectus

Straight.

650. serrated

Saw-toothed.

651. somite

An embryonic segment of mesoderm.

652. synergist

A muscle that works with a prime mover.

653. synergy

Coordination between agonist and antagonist that produces smooth movements.

654. triceps

Three-headed muscle.

655. trismus

A tetanic jaw muscle spasm.

656. voluntary

Under conscious control.

Physiology of Nerve Tissue

657. **absolute refractory period**

Period after stimulation during which a neuron cannot be stimulated no matter how strong the stimulus.

658. **acetylcholine**

A neurotransmitter released by many axons, especially those that control skeletal muscles.

659. **action potential**

Wave of change in electrical potential across the cell membrane of an excited cell; impulse.

660. **action potential with plateau**

A flat, prolonged potential seen in certain smooth muscle cells.

661. **all-or-none law**

The general idea that if a neuron responds to a stimulus it conducts a signal at maximum strength.

662. **axoaxonic synapse**

A site at which an axon of one neuron relays a signal to an axon of another neuron.

663. **axodendritic synapse**

A very common site at which an axon of one neuron relays a signal to a dendrite of another neuron.

664. **axon**

The part of a neuron that typically carries impulses away from the cell body toward another neuron.

665. **axon terminal**

The end of an axon from which neurotransmitter is released.

666. axosomatic synapse

A site at which an axon of one neuron relays a signal to the cell body of another neuron.

667. bipolar neuron

Neuron with axon and dendrites extending in opposite directions from the cell body.

668. catecholamine

A class of amines that act as chemical messengers; dopamine, epinephrine, and norepinephrine.

669. cholinergic

Relating to a neuron whose terminals release acetylcholine.

670. cholinesterase

An enzyme that degrades acetylcholine.

671. cholinesterase inhibitor

A substance that blocks cholinesterase action.

672. chromatolysis

Breakdown of chromatin.

673. conductivity

Ability to relay an electrical impulse.

674. convergence

Coming together.

675. dendrite

A cytoplasmic process of a neuron that commonly receives signals from other neurons.

676. **dendrodendritic synapse**

A rare neuronal junction in which a dendrite of one neuron relays signals to a dendrite of another neuron.

677. **depolarization**

Loss of negative charge inside a cell usually associated with the transmission of a nerve impulse.

678. **divergence**

Radiating out in different directions.

679. **dopamine**

A neurotransmitter and precursor of norepinephrine.

680. **ependymal cells**

Neuroglia cells found in the lining of brain ventricles and the central canal of the spinal cord.

681. **excitatory postsynaptic potential (EPSP)**

A potential resulting from partial depolarization of a postsynaptic neuron.

682. **glioma**

Tumor of neuroglial cells.

683. **inhibitory postsynaptic potential (IPSP)**

A potential that hyperpolarizes a postsynaptic membrane.

684. **internodal**

Between nodes.

685. **membrane potential**

An electrical potential (potential difference between) the inside and outside of a membrane.

686. microglia

Small supporting cells of the central nervous system.

687. motor nerve

Nerve that carries impulses from the central nervous system to an effector.

688. motor neuron

A neuron that carries impulses toward a muscle or gland.

689. multipolar neuron

Neuron with one axon and numerous dendrites.

690. myelin

An insulating substance deposited around axons.

691. myelin sheath

Insulating layer that protects most nerves.

692. myelinated

Having myelin.

693. nerve fiber

Axon or dendrite of a neuron.

694. neurilemma

The Schwann cell membrane.

695. neuroglia

Supporting cells of the nervous system.

696. neuroglial

Related to supporting cells of the nervous system.

697. neuromuscular junction

Region where a motor neuron interacts with the membrane of a skeletal muscle cell.

698. neuronal pool

A complex set of central nervous system synapses.

699. neuropeptide

A molecule made of a chain of amino acids that influences neural function.

700. neurotransmitter

A chemical substance from one neuron that transmits a signal to another neuron at a synapse.

701. neurulation

Formation of a neural tube as a part of embryonic development.

702. Nissl granule

Granules containing RNA and endoplasmic reticulum in nerve cell bodies and dendrites.

703. node of Ranvier

A gap in an axon's myelin sheath.

704. noradrenalin

Norepinephrine.

705. norepinephrine

A neurotransmitter of the sympathetic division of the autonomic nervous system and of some brain neurons.

706. oligodendrocyte

Myelin-producing cell of the central nervous system.

707. perikaryon

Substance around a nucleus; the cell body of a neuron.

708. polarized

State of a resting membrane that allows it to respond to a stimulus.

709. postsynaptic

Referring to a neuron that receives a neurotransmitter at a synapse.

710. presynaptic

Referring to a neuron that releases a neurotransmitter at a synapse.

711. principle of forward conduction

A rule that signals travel along axons toward the next neuron in a pathway.

712. relative refractory period

Period after stimulation during which a neuron responds only to a strong stimulus.

713. Schwann cell

A myelin producing cell in the peripheral nervous system.

714. sensory nerve

Nerve that carries impulses to the central nervous system.

715. sensory neuron

Neuron that initiates nerve impulses as a result of being stimulated.

716. soma

Cell body.

717. synapse

A junction where a signal passes from one neuron to the next in a pathway, usually by neurotransmitter diffusion.

718. synaptic

Of a synapse.

719. synaptic cleft

Fluid-filled space between two neurons across which a neurotransmitter diffuses.

720. synaptic delay

Time for a neurotranmsitter to diffuse across a synapse and initiate a postsynaptic impulse.

721. unipolar neuron

Neuron having only one process made from fusion of two processes.

722. Wallerian degeneration

Axon disintegration in an injured neuron distal to the point of injury.

723. white matter

Myelinated nerve fibers of the central nervous system.

Central Nervous System

724. afferent

Movement toward a structure.

725. alpha wave

A brain wave that occurs in an awake, relaxed state.

726. Alzheimer's disease

A degenerative neurological disorder associated with memory loss and behavioral changes.

727. amygdaloid

Almond-shaped.

728. anencephaly

Absence of a brain.

729. anesthetic

Agent that produces temporary loss of sensation.

730. aqueduct

A canal that conducts liquid.

731. arachnoid

Spiderlike, as the delicate middle meninges that covers the brain and spinal cord.

732. arbor vitae

Treelike pattern of cerebellar white matter.

733. association fiber

A neural tract that relays impulses between parts of the cerebrum.

734. association neuron

A neuron that relays impulses from sensory to motor neurons, especially in the spinal cord.

735. astrocyte

A star-shaped neuroglial cell in the central nervous system.

736. Babinski reflex

A reflex of dorsiflexion of the toes when the sole of the foot is scratched.

737. basal nucleus

One of several aggregations of cell bodies deep in the base of the cerebrum.

738. beta wave

A brain wave that occurs during mental alertness.

739. blood-brain barrier

A specialized capillary structure that limits movement of substances from blood into brain tissue.

740. brain stem

Brain parts that relay impulses to and from the cerebrum, cerebellum, and other brain structures.

741. brain wave

An electrical signal detected on the scalp that represents brain activity.

742. Broca's motor speech area

A functional area of the cerebrum where thoughts are translated into speech.

743. Brown-Sequard syndrome

Partial paralysis in patients with injury to one side of the spinal cord.

744. cauda equina

A bundle of spinal nerve roots extending posteriorly from the end of the spinal cord; literally, horse's tail.

745. caudate nucleus

An aggregate of cell bodies deep within the cerebrum.

746. central nervous system (CNS)

Brain and spinal cord.

747. cerebellar

Relating to the cerebellum.

748. cerebellum

A brain component behind the cerebrum and above the pons concerned with the coordination of movements.

749. cerebral

Relating to the cerebrum.

750. cerebral aqueduct

Passage within the midbrain that connects the third and fourth ventricles.

751. cerebral cortex

Outer gray matter of the cerebrum.

752. cerebrospinal fluid

A clear fluid in spaces within and around the central nervous system.

753. cerebrovascular

Relating to blood vessels of the brain.

754. cerebrum

The largest brain component; responds to sensory impulses and carries out mental processes.

755. choroid plexus

One of several projections of vascular tissue that secrete cerebrospinal fluid into brain ventricles.

756. cingulate

Relating to a bundle of fibers.

757. circle of Willis

A ring of blood vessels at the base of the brain by which blood reaches alternate circulatory pathways in the brain.

758. command neuron

Interneuron in an extrapyramidal nucleus that participates in regulation of motor circuits of the spinal cord.

759. commissural fiber

A nerve fiber in a bundle that connects the left and right sides of the brain and spinal cord.

760. consciousness

Awareness of signals from the sense organs.

761. contralateral

On the opposite side.

762. conus medullaris

The posterior end of the spinal cord.

763. corpus callosum

An aggregation of myelinated neural fibers that carry impulses between the two cerebral hemispheres.

764. cortex

Outer portion of an organ; literally, bark.

765. decussate

Cross the midline of the body.

766. delta wave

A brain wave that occurs mainly during deep sleep.

767. diencephalon

Embryonic brain region between the cerebrum and midbrain; develops into thalamus, hypothalamus, and third ventricle.

768. dura mater

The tough outermost meninges that surrounds the brain, spinal cord, and other meninges.

769. dural

Of the dura mater.

770. dyslexia

Inability to read with understanding, often because of reversals of letters in words.

771. efferent

Leading away from.

772. electroencephalogram (EEG)

A record of electrical changes detected on the scalp and associated with brain activity.

773. emotion

A state of feeling; the affective aspect of consciousness.

774. encephalitis

Inflammation of the brain.

775. endogenous

Originating within an organism.

776. epidural

Outside the dura mater.

777. exogenous

Originating outside the body.

778. extrapyramidal tract

Bundle of motor fibers in the spinal cord that does not pass through the pyramids.

779. filum terminale

Fibrous attachment of the spinal cord to the coccyx.

780. forebrain

Early embryonic portion of the brain that gives rise to the telencephalon and diencephalon.

781. funiculus

Bundle of fibers in a spinal cord tract; white matter.

782. gamma-aminobutyric acid (GABA)

An inhibitory neurotrasmitter from some neurons of the central nervous system.

783. graded potential

A local change in a membrane potential proportional to the strength of a stimulus.

784. gray matter

Unmyelinated tissue (mainly cell bodies) in the central nervous system.

785. gyrus

A fold, such as a convolution of the cerebrum.

786. habit-forming

A property that causes some people to make great effort to obtain a drug.

787. habituation

Gradual adaptation to a continuing stimulus.

788. hemisection

Cutting through the tracts in one side of the spinal cord.

789. hippocampal

Of the hippocampus.

790. hippocampus

A part of the limbic system in the temporal region and concerned with emotion and memory.

791. hydrocephalus

Excessive cerebrospinal fluid in brain ventricles; water on the brain.

792. hypoglossal

Under the tongue.

793. innate

Already present at birth.

794. innervation

Nerve supply.

795. internal capsule

Band of fibers (white matter) between basal nuclei and the thalamus.

796. interneuron

A neuron that relays impulses between a sensory and a motor neuron, typically found in the spinal cord.

797. ipsilateral

On the same side.

798. lateralization

Functional variation in the two sides of a bilateral structure, especially the cerebrum.

799. learning

A behavioral change in response to external stimuli.

800. limbic system

A part of the brain mainly associated with emotions.

801. locus ceruleus

A nucleus of the reticular formation concerned with the regulation of sleep and wakefulness.

802. manic-depressive psychosis

A severe mental disorder characterized wide mood swings.

803. medulla

The inner core of an organ.

804. medulla oblongata

A part of the brain continuous with the spinal cord.

805. meninges

Membranes that surround the brain and spinal cord.

806. mesencephalon

A region of the embryonic brain near the middle of the brain.

807. midbrain

Brain stem region between diencephalon and pons.

808. multiple sclerosis

A central nervous system disease in which tissue hardens and fails to relay impulses.

809. myelencephalon

Hindbrain, especially the medulla oblongata.

810. myelomeningocele

Birth defect in which part of the spinal cord and its meninges protrude from the vertebral column.

811. neocortex

The most recently evolved part of the cerebrum.

812. neural crest

Cells that give rise to sensory neurons, adrenal medulla, and the autonomic nervous system.

813. neural tube

A tube formed by invagination of ectoderm that produces to the nervous system.

814. neurofibrillary tangles

Masses of disorderly neural fibers in the brains of Alzheimer patients.

815. Parkinson's disease

Muscle rigidity and tremors because of dopamine deficiency in the brain.

816. peduncle

One of several tracts that connect structures within the brain.

817. physiological dependence

The need for a drug to prevent withdrawal symptoms.

818. pia mater

A delicate membrane on the surface of the brain and spinal cord.

819. pineal gland

A gland between the cerebral hemispheres associated with regulating circadian rhythms.

820. pons

A part of the brain stem associated with the cerebellum.

821. pontine

Relating to the pons.

822. projection fiber

A fiber that connects the cerebral cortex with other central nervous system components.

823. prosencephalon

An anterior part of the embryonic brain.

824. Purkinje cell

A cerebellar neuron that synapses with a very large number of other cells.

825. putamen

Part of the basal nuclei of the cerebrum.

826. pyramid

A cone-shaped prominence on an organ.

827. pyramidal tract

Motor fibers passing through the medullary pyramids that control voluntary movements.

828. quadrate

Four-sided.

829. rapid-eye-movement (REM) sleep

Sleep interval in which the eyeballs move and the EEG resembles wakefulness; paradoxical sleep.

830. red nucleus

A midbrain nucleus from which the rubrospinal tract arises.

831. reticular activating system (RAS)

A brain stem structure involved in maintaining consciousness.

832. reticular formation

Structure in the brain stem that regulates sensory input to the cerebral cortex.

833. rhinencephalon

Part of cerebrum concerned with olfactory impulses.

834. rhombencephalon

A posterior part of the embryonic brain.

835. schizophrenia

A mental disorder involving a complex set of disturbances in thinking and feeling.

836. seasonal affective disorder (SAD)

Depression attributed to lessened light in fall and winter.

837. serotonin

A substance secreted as a brain neurotransmitter and a gut hormone.

838. spinal nerve

One of 31 pairs of nerves that carry impulses between the spinal cord and other body parts.

839. spinal reflex

Somatic reflex facilitated by impulses going to and from the spinal cord.

840. subarachnoid

Beneath the arachnoid membrane.

841. subconscious

Partially conscious.

842. subdural

Beneath the dura mater.

843. substantia nigra

A nucleus of pigmented cells; one of the basal nuclei.

844. subthalamic

Beneath the thalamus.

845. tardive dyskinesia

Involuntary movements probobly caused by long-term treatment with tranquilizers.

846. telencephalon

Anterior part of forebrain which gives rise to olfactory lobes and cerebral cortex.

847. thalamus

Subcortical gray matter near the anterior end of the brain stem.

848. theta wave

A brain wave that occurs in children and in some adults with brain disorders.

849. tolerance

A condition in which need for larger doses develops to get the same effect.

850. tract

A bundle of myelinated neurons in the brain or spinal cord.

851. vermis

Worm; a part of the cerebellum.

Somatic Nervous System

852. bilateral

Relating to both sides of the body; having left and right sides.

853. brachial

Of the arm.

854. cranial nerve

One of twelve pairs of nerves that arise from the brain and carry impulses to and from it.

855. endoneurium

Connective tissue around individual nerve fibers.

856. epineurium

Connective tissue forming a protective cover over an entire nerve.

857. extrafusal

Outside a muscle spindle.

858. ganglion

An aggregation of cell bodies in the peripheral nervous system.

859. Golgi tendon organ

A proprioceptor located in a tendon.

860. intrafusal

Modified muscle fibers that detect stretching within a muscle spindle.

861. kinesthetic

Concerned with sensing movement.

862. lumbosacral

Of the lower back and sacral regions.

863. mixed nerve

A nerve with both sensory and motor fibers.

864. muscle spindle

A spindle-shaped proprioceptor in a skeletal muscle.

865. nerve

A bundle of axons covered with a connective tissue sheaths.

866. neural oscillator

A process that control behaviors such as repetitive movements.

867. neuralgia

Pain related to a nerve.

868. neuritis

Inflammation of a nerve.

869. paraplegia

Paralysis of the legs and lower body.

870. pattern generator

A control mechanism for repetitive movements.

871. perineurium

A connective tissue sheath covering a bundle of nerve fibers.

872. plexus

A network, usually of nerves or blood vessels.

873. poliomyelitis

Inflammation and sometimes destruction of motor cells in the anterior horn of the spinal cord.

874. proprioceptor

Any sensory receptor in a muscle, joint, or tendon that detects position or movement.

875. quadriplegia

Paralysis of all four limbs.

876. reciprocal innervation

A set of neural connections that can slow one process and accelerate another.

877. rete

Network.

878. root

A base or foundation.

879. sciatic

Of the hip.

880. somatic

Of the body.

881. spinal shock

A temporary condition after a spinal injury during which spinal reflexes inferior to the injury are lost.

882. stretch reflex

Muscle contraction following stimulation of stretch receptors in a muscle or its tendon.

883. subneural

Beneath a nerve.

884. tendon organ

A sensory receptor that responds to stretching of a tendon.

885. withdrawal reflex

A reflex that leads to flexion and removal of a limb from a painful stimulus.

Autonomic Nervous System

886. adrenergic

Concerning a neuron that releases norepinephrine (adrenalin).

887. autonomic nervous system

A nervous system component that regulates internal organ functions and involuntary processes.

888. beta blocker

A drug that interferes with sympathetic signals that would ordinarily stimulate beta receptors.

889. biofeedback

Use of signals about levels of autonomic processes to control those processes.

890. craniosacral

Of the cranial and sacral regions.

891. dual innervation

Having both sympathetic and parasympathetic innervation in an organ.

892. parasympathetic division

Autonomic component that accelerates digestion and other functions not essential to a response to stress.

893. parasympatholytic

Concerning substances that block or counteract sympathetic signals.

894. parasympathomimetic

Concerning substances that mimic parasympathetic nervous system action.

895. postganglionic

Concerning a neuron that receives signals across a synapse in a ganglion; second neuron in an autonomic pathway.

896. preganglionic

Concerning a neuron that sends signals across a synapse in a ganglion; first neuron in an autonomic pathway.

897. splanchnic

Of the viscera.

898. sympathetic chain ganglion

An aggregation of the cell bodies of postsynaptic neurons of the sympathetic division.

899. sympathetic division

The part of the autonomic nervous system that can respond to stressful situations.

900. sympathetic tone

Partial vasoconstriction maintained by sympathetic signals.

901. sympatholytic

Blocking or counteracting sympathetic signals.

902. sympathomimetic

Mimicking the action of the sympathetic division, or a drug that does so.

903. thoracolumbar

Of the chest and lumbar regions.

904. vasomotor fiber

Sympathetic nerve fiber that carries impulses to control smooth muscle in blood vessel walls.

Sensory Organs

905. **acceleratory reflex**

A reflex that maintains balance during starting, stopping, and turning motions.

906. **accommodation**

Adjustment of the focal distance of the eyes to see close objects clearly.

907. **adaptation**

Decrease in excitability of sensory receptors after a period of continuous, constant intensity stimulation.

908. **amplitude**

Signal strength; the intensity of a sound.

909. **ampulla**

A dilation in a passageway.

910. **aqueous**

Watery.

911. **aqueous humor**

Clear fluid in the anterior chambers of the eye.

912. **arrestin**

A protein that blocks binding of opsin to transducin in the dark.

913. **astigmatism**

Blurred vision due to irregular curvature of one or more refractive surfaces in the eye.

914. attenuation

Lessening of an effect.

915. auditory

Of hearing.

916. auditory ossicle

Any of the three small bones that conduct sound vibrations through the middle ear.

917. baroreceptor

Pressure detector.

918. basilar membrane

Inner ear membrane associated with sound receptors.

919. binocular vision

Sight using two eyes that allows perception of three-dimensionality.

920. blind spot

Region of the retina that lacks light receptors where optic nerve fibers leave the eye.

921. canal of Schlemm

Passageway in the anterior eye that drains aqueous humor to the nasal cavity.

922. cataract

Opacity of the eye lens.

923. cerumen

Earwax.

924. ceruminous

Concerning earwax or glands that secrete it.

925. chemoreceptor

A receptor that responds to certain chemical substances.

926. chiasma

A site at which fibers cross over.

927. chlorolabe

A cone pigment that absorbs green light.

928. choroid

Vascular middle layer of the eyeball.

929. ciliary body

Anteriormost part of the choroid layer, which contains ciliary muscles that participate in accommodation.

930. cochlea

Snail-shaped bony part of the inner ear.

931. cochlear

Of the cochlea.

932. conduction deafness

Loss of hearing by failure of vibrations being transmitted to sound receptors.

933. cone

A light receptor that responds to a certain color.

934. conjunctiva

A mucous membrane lining the eyelids and covering the anterior eyeball surface.

935. cornea

A transparent part of the anterior eye surface.

936. cupula

A domelike cup-shaped structure.

937. cyanolabe

A cone pigment that responds to blue light.

938. decibel

A unit on the logarithmic scale of sound intensity.

939. diopter

A measure of the strength of a lens in bending light.

940. dynorphin

A polypeptide related to an enkephalin.

941. emmetropia

Normal vision, neither near- nor farsighted.

942. endorphin

A peptide that binds to opiate receptors in the brain.

943. enkephalin

A peptide derived from endorphin that binds to opiate receptors in the brain.

944. enteric

Of the intestine.

945. erythrolabe

A cone pigment sensitive to red light.

946. exteroceptor

A sensory receptor that detects environmental changes.

947. fibrous tunic

Outer layer of the eye.

948. focal length

Distance from lens to point at which light focuses behind it.

949. focal point

Point where light rays passing through a lens focus, or converge, behind it.

950. fovea centralis

A pit in the retina that contains only cone receptors; region of greatest visual acuity.

951. frequency

Number of occurrences of an event in a give period, such as vibrations per second of sound waves.

952. generator potential

The potential produced by initial depolarization of a sensory receptor.

953. geniculate

Bent, like a knee.

954. glaucoma

A disorder in which aqueous humor accumulates and exerts excessive intraocular pressure.

955. gustation

Sense of taste.

956. gustatory

Pertaining to the sense of taste.

957. hair cell

A sensory receptor that is stimulated by movement of fluid.

958. heliocotrema

A helix; a passage at the tip of the cochlea between the scala tympani and the scala vestibuli.

959. hertz

A unit of vibration frequency.

960. humor

Fluid.

961. hypermetropia

Farsightedness.

962. intensity

Degree of activity or tension.

963. interoreceptor

Sensory receptor in a visceral organ.

964. iris

Muscular diaphragm anterior to the eye lens that regulates the amount of light entering the eye.

965. isthmus

Constriction; neck.

966. labyrinth

Maze.

967. lacrimal

Of tears.

968. lateral inhibition

Suppression of hair cells adjacent to those stimulated, which makes signals from stimulated receptors clearer.

969. law of adequate stimulus

A law stating that a receptor responds only if it receives a sufficiently strong stimulus.

970. lens

Transparent, biconcave structure behind the iris that focuses eye on far or near objects by changing shape.

971. lysozyme

An enzyme in tears that can destroy microbes.

972. macula

An inner ear structure that contains sensory receptors for static equilibrium.

973. mechanoreceptor

A receptor that responds to mechanical pressure.

974. Meniere's disease

A semicircular canal inflammation that leads to sight, hearing, and balance disorders.

975. meridional fibers

Muscle fibers that attach the suspensory ligament to choroid layer and regulate ligament length.

976. migraine

Affecting half of the head.

977. modiolus

A structure that supports the cochlea.

978. motion sickness

A disturbance in semicircular canal function resulting from changes in motion.

979. myopia

Nearsightedness.

980. naloxone

A drug that competes for receptors and counteracts opiate overdoses.

981. nerve deafness

Hearing impairment due to damage to sound receptors or nerve fibers leading from them to the brain.

982. nociceptor

A receptor that responds specifically to painful stimuli.

983. olfaction

Sense of smell.

984. olfactory

Of the sense of smell.

985. olfactory epithelium

Lining of nasal cavity that contains smell receptors.

986. ophthalmic

Of the eye.

987. opsin

A protein that combines with retinine in the retina.

988. optic

Of the eye or concerning the properties of light.

989. optic chiasma

A site anterior to the pituitary where medial fibers of each optic nerve cross from one side of the body to the other.

990. optic disk

Region of the retina lacking receptors where optic nerve fibers leave the eyeball; blind spot.

991. organ of Corti

The inner ear structure where sound receptors are located.

992. otolith

A small calcium carbonate particle in a receptor for static equilibrium; an ear stone.

993. oval window

A membrane-covered opening from the middle to the inner ear across which the stapes transmits vibrations.

994. Pacinian corpuscle

A receptor that responds to pressure.

995. palpebra

Eyelid.

996. perception

Conscious interpretation of information from sensory receptors.

997. perilymph

A clear fluid in the osseous labyrinth, which surrounds the membranous labyrinth in the inner ear.

998. phantom pain

Pain felt as if it originated in a body part no longer present, such as an amputated limb.

999. photon

The smallest unit of light energy.

1000. photoreceptor

A receptor that responds to light.

1001. pinna

The flap-like part of the ear projecting from the head.

1002. pitch

A sound quality determined by vibration frequency.

1003. presbyopia

Loss of lens accommodation, and thus close-up vision; literally, elder vision.

1004. pressoreceptor

Sensory receptor that detects pressure changes.

1005. pupil

Opening in the iris through which light enters the eye.

1006. rarefaction

Decreased density.

1007. receptor potential

Graded potential across the membrane of a sensory receptor.

1008. referred pain

Pain felt as if it came from a site other than its actual origin.

1009. refraction

Bending of light rays as they pass from a medium of one density to a medium of a different density.

1010. retina

The innermost layer of the eye, which contains light receptors.

1011. retinene

A carotenoid pigment that binds to opsin.

1012. rhodopsin

A light-sensitive protein found in rods of the retina.

1013. rod

A receptor in the retina that responds to different intensities of light but not to color.

1014. round window

A membrane-covered opening between the middle and inner ear.

1015. saccadic

Movements of the eyeball in the course of following a moving object.

1016. saccule

A little sac, as in the vestibule of the inner ear.

1017. scala tympani

The inferior canal of the cochlea.

1018. scala vestibuli

The superior canal of the cochlea.

1019. sclera

Outer fibrous layer of the eyeball.

1020. semicircular canal

One of three pairs of fluid-filled inner ear passageways that detect head movements.

1021. sensation

An impression conveyed.

1022. sensory

Concerned with sensation.

1023. sensory receptor

Dendrite or other cell part that can respond to a stimulus.

1024. special sense

Any of the following senses: taste, smell, vision, hearing, and equilibrium.

1025. static equilibrium

Maintenance of balance while the head is stationary.

1026. suspensory

Serving to hold up.

1027. taste bud

A structure on the tongue containing taste receptor cells.

1028. tear

A fluid released from tear glands.

1029. tectorial membrane

A membrane overlying the hair cells in the organ of Corti.

1030. thermoreceptor

A receptor that detects temperature changes.

1031. timbre

A sound quality based on a tone and its overtones.

1032. tinnitus

Ringing in the ears.

1033. transducin

Enzyme involved in visual process.

1034. transduction

The conversion of a signal from one type to another, such as from chemical to electrical.

1035. tympanic membrane

Eardrum; membrane between the external and middle ear.

1036. utricle

Large chamber in the ear vestibule that contains receptors for equilibrium.

1037. uvea

The middle layer of the eyeball.

1038. vestibular

Of a vestibule.

1039. vestibule

A space or cavity near the entrance of a canal.

1040. visceroceptor

A receptor in or near an internal organ.

1041. visual area

A region of the occipital lobe of the cerebrum that receives and processes signals from the retina.

1042. vitreous

Glassy.

The Endocrine System

1043. adenohypophysis

Anterior pituitary gland.

1044. adrenal

Above the kidney; a gland lying superior to the kidney.

1045. adrenalin

A hormone secreted by the adrenal medulla; epinephrine.

1046. adrenocorticotropic hormone

A hormone that stimulates the adrenal cortex to secrete hormones.

1047. alarm reaction

The body's characteristic response to a stressful situation.

1048. aldosterone

An adrenocortical hormone that increases reabsorption of sodium.

1049. anabolic steroid

A synthetic hormone that increases muscle size.

1050. androgen

A molecule with male hormone activity.

1051. angiotensin

A substance that causes vasoconstriction and aldosterone release.

1052. angiotensinogen

Inactive precursor of angiotensin.

1053. antidiuretic hormone (ADH)

A hypothalamic hormone stored in the posterior pituitary gland that stimulates water conservation by the kidneys.

1054. atrial natriuretic hormone (ANH)

A substance secreted by the atria that accelerates sodium excretion in the kidneys.

1055. beta lipotropin

A molecule from which endorphins are derived.

1056. calcitonin

A hormone that lowers blood calcium.

1057. calmodulin

An intracellular calcium carrier molecule.

1058. corticosterone

A steroid hormone from adrenal cortex.

1059. cortisol

An adrenocortical hormone that helps regulate carbohydrate metabolism and counteracts inflammation.

1060. cyclic AMP

Intracellular second messenger that mediates effects of hormones at receptors on the cell membrane.

1061. diabetes insipidus

A disorder in which a lack of antidiuretic hormone lead to production of large quantities of dilute urine.

1062. diffuse endocrine system (DES)

Assortment of hormone-secreting cells in various locations throughout the body.

1063. endocrine

Concerning a ductless gland.

1064. epinephrine

Main hormone from the adrenal medulla.

1065. eustress

A productive kind of stress.

1066. exhaustion stage

Stage of stress at which the body has failed to cope.

1067. follicle-stimulating hormone (FSH)

A hormone that stimulates maturation of ova and sperm.

1068. gastrin

A hormone from the stomach lining that circulates in the blood and stimulates HCl secretion.

1069. general adaptation syndrome

A set of changes that occur in animals under stress.

1070. glucagon

A hormone that raises blood glucose.

1071. glucocorticoid

A hormone that helps to regulate carbohydrate metabolism.

1072. gonadotropin

Hormone from the anterior pituitary gland that stimulates gonads.

1073. growth hormone

Hormone from the anterior pituitary gland that stimulates growth and maintains adult body size.

1074. hormone

A regulatory substance from an endocrine cell that is transported in the blood to its target cells.

1075. human chorionic gonadotropin

A placental hormone that stimulates the corpus luteum to secrete hormones.

1076. hypophysis

The pituitary gland.

1077. hypothalamus

A part of the brain that connects and serves both the nervous and endocrine systems.

1078. insulin

A hormone from the pancreas that causes cells to take in glucose and stimulates protein synthesis.

1079. islet of Langerhans

Cluster of hormone-secreting cells in the pancreas.

1080. luteinizing hormone (LH)

A hormone that helps to cause ovulation and other reproductive processes.

1081. mineralocorticoid

A hormone that regulates mineral metabolism.

1082. natriuresis

Stimulation of sodium excretion.

1083. neurohypophysis

The posterior, neural part of the pituitary gland.

1084. oxytocin

A hormone from the hypothalamus that stimulates uterine contractions and milk let down.

1085. parathormone

A hormone from the parathyorid gland that decreases blood calcium.

1086. parathyroid glands

Glands imbedded in the thyorid gland that produce a hormone important in calcium metabolism.

1087. pituitary gland

Neuroendocrine gland at base of brain, which provides connection between nervous and endocrine functions.

1088. portal

Concerning blood circulation from one set of capillaries to another, as between the hypothalamus and pituitary.

1089. progesterone

A hormone that helps to maintain pregnancy.

1090. prolactin

A hormone that stimulates milk secretion.

1091. prostaglandin

A substance derived from the fatty acid arachidonic acid that acts over short distances as a chemical messenger.

1092. puberty

A period during which sexual maturity is achieved.

1093. radioimmunoassay

Measurement of a substance's concentration using antibodies that bind to it and emit radiation.

1094. Rathke's pouch

An embryonic structure from which the anterior pituitary develops.

1095. relaxin

A hormone from the corpus luteum released during pregnancy.

1096. resistance stage

A period during which the body successfully copes with stress.

1097. second messenger

Intracellular substance that relays a signal from an extracellular substance bound to a membrane receptor.

1098. somatostatin

Growth-hormone inhibiting hormone.

1099. somatotropin

Growth hormone.

1100. stress

A condition produced by a variety of injurious agents that affects many body systems.

1101. stressor

An agent or event that produces stress.

1102. target cell

A cell that can respond to a certain hormone.

1103. testosterone

A male hormone.

1104. thymosin

A hormone secreted by the thymus gland.

1105. thymus gland

A gland that processes and activates T lymphocytes before it regresses during puberty.

1106. thyroid gland

A gland in the throat that produces hormones important in regulating the metabolic rate.

1107. thyroid-stimulating hormone (TSH)

A hormone that stimulates hormone secretion by the thyroid gland.

1108. tropic

Influencing another organ or process.

1109. vasopressin

Antidiuretic hormone.

1110. zona fasciculata

Middle layer of cells in the adrenal cortex.

1111. zona glomerulosa

Outer layer of cells in the adrenal cortex.

1112. zona reticularis

Inner layer of cells in the adrenal cortex.

Blood and Lymph

1113. agranular leukocyte

A white blood cell lacking cytoplasmic granules.

1114. albumin

A small protein made in the liver and released into blood.

1115. anemia

A hemoglobin deficiency associated with too few erythrocytes or poorly functioning ones.

1116. anticoagulant

A substance the prevents blood from clotting.

1117. antithrombin

Substance in plasma that inhibits coagulation by neutralizing thrombin.

1118. aplastic

Having no tendency to undergo cell division.

1119. apoferritin

A protein that carries iron.

1120. basophil

A leukocyte with granular cytoplasm stainable by a basic dye.

1121. bilirubin

A red bile pigment from hemoglobin breakdown.

1122. biliverdin

A green bile pigment from hemoglobin breakdown.

1123. blood

Fluid pumped by the heart through a closed system of vessels.

1124. Bohr effect

Tendency of a high oxygen concentration in the lungs to facilitate release of carbon dioxide from hemoglobin.

1125. carbaminohemoglobin

Hemoglobin to which carbon dioxide is bound.

1126. cardiovascular

Of the heart and blood vessels.

1127. ceruloplasmin

A blood protein that transports copper.

1128. cisterna chyli

Large lymphatic vessel that drains lymph from the abdominal organs and legs.

1129. clot retraction

Shrinkage of a blood clot.

1130. coumarin

An anticoagulant that blocks synthesis of some clotting factors in the liver.

1131. cross-matching

Comparison of donor and prospective recipient bloods to detect possibilities of agglutination.

1132. diapedesis

Squeezing of leukocytes between the cells of capillary walls.

1133. differential white cell count

Determination of relative numbers of different kinds of leukocytes in a blood sample.

1134. edema

Excess fluid accumulation in the tissues.

1135. embolus

A blood clot traveling in a blood vessel.

1136. endolymph

Fluid located in the membranous labyrinth of the inner ear.

1137. eosinophil

A granular leukocyte stained by the dye eosin.

1138. erythrocyte

Red blood cell.

1139. erythropoiesis

Process of red blood cell formation.

1140. erythropoietin

A substance from the kidney that stimulates erythropoiesis.

1141. ferritin

A molecule made up of the protein apoferritin and iron.

1142. fibrin

A fibrous protein that forms a network in a blood clot.

1143. fibrinogen

An inactive precursor of the protein fibrin.

1144. formed elements

Cells or cell fragments in blood.

1145. gastroferrin

An iron-binding protein that transports iron from the stomach lumen to mucosal cells.

1146. globin

A globular protein found in hemoglobin and certain other biological molecules.

1147. globulin

A globular protein, including many in the plasma.

1148. granular leukocyte

A white blood cell with granular cytoplasm.

1149. hematocrit

The proportion of erythrocytes in a volume of blood.

1150. hematopoiesis

The formation of blood cells.

1151. heme

An iron-containing pigment in hemoglobin that binds oxygen.

1152. hemocytoblast

Cell that gives rise to several kinds of blood cells.

1153. hemodialysis

The removal of substances from the blood by dialysis.

1154. hemoglobin

The oxygen-carrying protein in erythrocytes.

1155. hemolysis

Breakdown of erythrocytes with hemoglobin release.

1156. hemolytic

Concerning hemolysis.

1157. hemophilia

An inherited inability to produce a blood clotting factor.

1158. hemopoiesis

The formation of blood cells.

1159. hemopoietic

Related to hemopoiesis.

1160. hemosiderin

A molecule that binds and stores iron.

1161. hemostasis

The arrest of bleeding.

1162. heparin

An anticoagulant synthesized in several body tissues.

1163. hirudin

An anticoagulant secreted by leeches.

1164. jaundice

Yellowish tone to skin and membranes caused by excess bile pigments in the blood.

1165. leukemia

A malignant proliferation of leukocytes.

1166. leukocyte

A white blood cell.

1167. lymph

Interstitial fluid in a lymphatic vessel.

1168. lymphocyte

A leukocyte that participates in an immune response.

1169. monocyte

A large, phagocytic, agranular leukocyte.

1170. myeloid

Derived from bone marrow.

1171. neutrophil

A granular leukocyte not stained by either acidic or basic stains.

1172. oxyhemoglobin

Hemoglobin to which oxygen is bound.

1173. pernicious anemia

Anemia due to a lack of intrinsic factor and therefore vitamin B12.

1174. plasma

The fluid part of blood including inactive clotting factors.

1175. plasmin

An enzyme built into blood clots as they form that gradually dissolves them.

1176. plasminogen

Inactive plasmin.

1177. platelet

A megakaryocyte fragment in blood that participates in blood clotting reactions.

1178. polycythemia

An excess of erythrocytes.

1179. polymorphonuclear leukocyte (PMNL)

A white blood cell with an irregular, lobed nucleus.

1180. prothrombin

Inactive thrombin.

1181. reticulocyte

Immature erythrocyte.

1182. serum

The fluid part of blood after removal of formed elements and clotting factors.

1183. sickle cell anemia

An inherited anemia in which erythrocytes sickle under low oxygen conditions.

1184. spectrin

A protein that maintains flexibility of erythrocyte membranes.

1185. streptokinase

An enzyme that digests blood clots used to treat coronary occlusion.

1186. T lymphocyte

A thymus-processed lymphocyte that can differentiate into several kinds of T cells.

1187. thalassemia

An anemia caused by a deficiency of alpha or beta of chains hemoglobin.

1188. thrombin

An enzyme that activates fibrinogen to fibrin in the blood clotting mechanism.

1189. thrombocyte

A platelet.

1190. thrombocytopenia

A deficiency of platelets.

1191. thrombus

A blood clot that is stationary in a blood vessel wall.

1192. tissue plasminogen activator (tPA)

A substance secreted by many tissues that activates plasminogen to plasmin.

1193. tissue thromboplastin

A substance from injured tissue that initiates extrinsic blood clotting.

1194. transferrin

An iron-transport protein in plasma.

1195. vascular

Containing blood vessels.

The Heart

1196. antrum

A chamber or cavity.

1197. aorta

A large artery that carries blood from the left ventricle to other arteries of the systemic circulation.

1198. aortic

Of the aorta.

1199. arrhythmia

Abnormal rhythm in signal conduction through the heart.

1200. artificial pacemaker

A device that automatically stimulates the heart and maintains a regular heart rate.

1201. atrial

Of the atria of the heart.

1202. atrioventricular

Of an atrium and ventricle.

1203. atrioventricular bundle

Group of fibers that conduct impulses from the AV node to the right and left ventricles; bundle of His.

1204. atrioventricular node

Specialized conducting cells clustered at the junction of atrial and ventricular muscle.

1205. atrium

A chamber or entrance.

1206. auricle

An earlike appendage.

1207. autoregulation

Self-regulation.

1208. AV node

An aggregation of tissue in the atrioventricular septum that conducts signals to control the heart beat.

1209. bradycardia

A slower than normal heart rate.

1210. cardiac

Of the heart.

1211. cardiac output

Quantity of blood pumped out of a ventricle in one minute.

1212. cardiac tamponade

Compression of the heart by fluid accumulating in the pericardial sac.

1213. cardiologist

A physician who specialized in treating heart disease.

1214. chordae tendineae

Tough connective tissue bands that attach A-V valve cusps to papillary muscles within the heart's ventricles.

1215. chronotropic

Time-related effects.

1216. circus rhythm

A circular or repetitive motion.

1217. conduction system

Fibers in heart muscle in which signals coordinate atrial and ventricular contractions.

1218. coronary

Of the heart; circling like a crown.

1219. defibrillation

Termination of an extremely fast heart rate by application of a strong electrical current.

1220. diastole

Dilation; a period of relaxation between heart contractions.

1221. diastolic

Of diastole.

1222. ductus

A tube that usually carries a secretion; duct.

1223. ectopic

Not in the normal location.

1224. electrocardiogram (ECG)

A record of electrical changes detected on the body surface associated with heart contractions.

1225. end-diastolic volume

Blood volume in a ventricle at the end of its relaxation period.

1226. endocarditis

Inflammation of the lining of the heart.

1227. endocardium

The heart's epithelial lining.

1228. epicardium

A connective tissue that covers the heart and lines the pericardial sac.

1229. fibrillation

Uncoordinated contraction of a small group of muscle fibers.

1230. flutter

Extremely rapid, ineffective contractions.

1231. Frank-Starling law

A law stating that stroke volume increases in proportion to stretching of muscle fibers in the heart.

1232. heart block

An arrhythmia due to disrupted conduction.

1233. heart murmur

An abnormal sound caused by turbulence around a defective valve.

1234. infarct

Region of damaged or dead cells resulting from diminished blood supply.

1235. interatrial

Between the atria of the heart.

1236. interventricular

Between the ventricles of the heart.

1237. isovolumetric

Having the same volume.

1238. left-to-right shunt

Abnormal blood flow from the left to the right side of the heart.

1239. mitral valve

A bicuspid valve between the left atrium and ventricle.

1240. myocardium

The thick muscular layer of the heart.

1241. pacemaker

An aggregation of cells that spontaneously excite other cells, as in the sinoatrial node.

1242. papillary muscles

Cardiac muscle extensions attached to chordae tendineae.

1243. pericardium

A sac around the heart.

1244. Purkinje fiber

The terminal ends of fibers in the heart's conduction system.

1245. QRS complex

A part of an electrocardiogram that appears as ventricles contract.

1246. right-to-left shunt

Abnormal blood flow directly from the right to the left side of the heart bypassing the pulmonary circuit.

1247. SA node

Part of the heart's conduction system that normally initiates contractions.

1248. semilunar

Shaped like a halfmoon.

1249. sinoatrial node

Cells specialized to conduct impulses in the wall of the right atrium; pacemaker.

1250. sinus bradycardia

A slow heart rate due to slow signaling by the SA node.

1251. sinus tachycardia

A rapid heart rate due to rapid signalling by the SA node.

1252. stenosis

Narrowing or constriction.

1253. stroke volume

Volume of blood ejected by one ventricle during a single contraction.

1254. systole

Contraction.

1255. systolic pressure

Pressure produced by contraction of a ventricle.

1256. T wave

A part of an electrocardiogram that occurs as ventricles repolarize.

1257. tachycardia

A rapid heart rate.

1258. tetralogy of Fallot

Four concurrent congenital heart defects.

1259. tricuspid

Having three points or cusps.

1260. valve

A structure in a passageway that prevents reflux.

1261. ventricle

A small cavity.

Blood Vessels and Lymphatics

1262. anastomosis

A connection between blood vessels or between nerves.

1263. aneurysm

A saclike dilation in an arterial wall.

1264. angiogenesis

Blood vessel development.

1265. angiogenic

Related to angiogenesis.

1266. angioplasty

Surgery on blood vessels.

1267. arteriogram

An image of an artery usually made by making X rays of opaque material in the artery.

1268. arteriole

A blood vessel between an artery and capillaries.

1269. artery

A large blood vessel carrying blood away from the heart.

1270. capacitance vessel

One of several vessels (veins) that together contain a large volume of blood.

1271. capillary

A small, thin blood vessel that connects an arteriole with a venule.

1272. celiac

Related to the abdomen.

1273. collateral circulation

Alternate pathways for the circulation of blood.

1274. endothelium

Epithelium that lines blood and lymph vessels.

1275. femoral

Of a femur.

1276. hemorrhoids

Enlarged mucosal blood vessels in the rectum.

1277. hepatic portal system

Blood vessels between capillaries of digestive system and those of the liver.

1278. lumen

Cavity inside a blood vessel, passage, or hollow organ.

1279. lymph node

A lymphatic tissue aggregation interposed at intervals along a lymphatic vessel.

1280. lymphatic

Concerning lymph or a vessel that carries it.

1281. lymphoid

Resembling lymph or lymphatic tissue.

1282. precapillary sphincter

Region in an arteriole that regulates blood flow through a capillary bed.

1283. sinusoid

A blood vessel similar to a capillary with a larger diameter.

1284. subclavian

Beneath the clavicle.

1285. thoracic duct

Large duct that receives lymph from whole body except for right arm and right side of head.

1286. thoroughfare channel

A capillary in a capillary that remains open continuously.

1287. umbilical cord

Structure containing arteries and veins that carry blood between a fetus and a placenta.

1288. varicose

Unnaturally swollen.

1289. varicosity

A condition with extreme swelling.

1290. vasa vasorum

Small blood vessels in the walls of larger blood vessels.

1291. vein

A blood vessel that carries blood to the heart.

1292. vena cava

A large vein that empties blood into the heart.

1293. venous

Of a vein.

1294. venule

A small vessel between capillaries and a vein.

Circulation & Circulatory Disorders

1295. angina pectoris

Severe, constrictive, suffocating chest pain associated with ischemic heart disease.

1296. arteriosclerosis

Any degenerative change that decreases the elasticity of an artery.

1297. atherosclerosis

Obstruction of arteries by hardened plaque deposits.

1298. blood pressure

Force blood exerts against a given area of vessel wall.

1299. cardioinhibitory

Having the effect of slowing the heart rate.

1300. carotid body

Structure at the branching of carotid arteries where chemoreceptors are located.

1301. carotid sinus

Dilation of a common carotid artery with receptors that help to regulate systemic blood pressure.

1302. central venous pressure

Pressure in veins near the heart.

1303. congestive heart failure

Loss of capacity to pump blood and associated accumulation of excess tissue fluids.

1304. embolism

Obstruction of a blood vessel by a moving clot or air bubble.

1305. essential hypertension

Elevated arterial blood pressure without a known cause.

1306. exchange vessel

Blood vessel through which substances are exchanged between blood and tissues; capillary.

1307. heart failure

Loss of ability to pump sufficient blood to supply body tissues with nutrients and remove wastes.

1308. hemorrhage

Loss of a significant volume of blood.

1309. hemorrhagic

Relating to a hemorrhage.

1310. hypertension

Excessively high blood pressure.

1311. hypotension

Excessively low blood pressure.

1312. hypovolemic

Having a subnormal volume.

1313. ischemia

Reduction in blood flow to an area.

1314. Korotkoff sound

A sound made by arterial blood heard through a stethoscope during measurement of blood pressure.

1315. laminar

Arranged in thin plates.

1316. mean arterial pressure (MAP)

Average pressure in an artery; diastolic pressure plus 1/3 the difference between systolic and diastolic pressures.

1317. myocardial infarction (MI)

Damage and sometimes death of heart muscle cells from interruption in blood supply.

1318. occlusion

Obstruction.

1319. oncotic pressure

Osmotic pressure created by the proteins and other molecules in a fluid.

1320. peripheral resistance

Degree to which friction between vessel walls and blood opposes flow.

1321. plaque

A sheetlike deposit.

1322. pressor

Factor that tends to increase pressure.

1323. pulse

Rhythmic expansion and contraction of an artery caused by the pumping action of the heart.

1324. pulse pressure

Difference between highest and lowest pressure in an artery caused by the heart's pumping action.

1325. resistance

Opposition to flow, as in blood vessels.

1326. resistance vessel

A blood vessel that resists stretching when under pressure; artery or arteriole.

1327. sphygmomanometer

A device used to measure blood pressure.

1328. stethoscope

An device used to amplify sounds from inside the body.

1329. stroke

Damage to brain tissue because of reduced blood supply; cerebrovascular accident.

1330. torr

A unit of pressure equal to that required to support a column of mercury 1 mm tall.

1331. vasoconstriction

Narrowing of the lumen of a blood vessel.

1332. vasodilation

Widening of the lumen of a blood vessel.

1333. vasomotor

Concerning the regulation of blood vessel diameter.

1334. vasomotor center

A region in the brain stem that regulates blood vessel diameters, especially in arterioles.

1335. viscosity

A fluid's tendency to resist flow.

Body Defense Mechanisms

1336. acquired immune deficiency syndrome (AIDS)

A viral disease that severely impairs immunity.

1337. acquired immunity

Disease resistance obtained from another's antibodies.

1338. active immunity

Disease resistance obtained by the immune system responding to a microorganism or a vaccine.

1339. agammaglobulinemia

An immunodeficiency due to a lack of B lymphocytes.

1340. agglutinin

An antibody in an agglutination reaction.

1341. agglutinogen

An antigen that elicits an agglutination reaction.

1342. allergen

A substance capable of eliciting an allergic reaction.

1343. allergy

Unusual sensitivity to a normally harmless concentration of substance.

1344. anaphylaxis

A severe allergic reaction to a substance after prior sensitization to it.

1345. antibody

A protein elicited by an antigen that can react with and inactivate the antigen.

1346. antigen

A substance that elicits a response from the immune system.

1347. antigen presenting cell

A macrophage or other cell that processes an antigen and presents it to a B or T lymphocyte.

1348. antigenic determinant

The part of an antigen molecule that elicits an immunologic response.

1349. antiviral protein

A protein produced by cells in response to stimulation by interferon.

1350. artificially acquired active immunity

Disease resistance obtained by stimulating the immune system with a vaccine.

1351. artificially acquired passive immunity

Temporary disease resistance obtained by receiving another's antibodies.

1352. atopy

A tendency to develop hypersensitivity and to produce large numbers of IgEs.

1353. autoantibody

An antibody against some substance normally present in the body.

1354. autoimmune disorder

A condition in which the body makes autoantibodies.

1355. autoimmune response

Release of effector T cells or antibodies that attack a person's own tissues.

1356. B lymphocyte

A lymphocyte that produces plasma cells, which in turn produce antibodies.

1357. blocking antibody

Antibody that binds to allergen and helps to prevent it from causing an allergic response.

1358. bursa of Fabricius

A structure found in birds where B lymphocyte differentiation was first identified.

1359. cell-mediated immunity

Disease resistance involving direct destruction of antigenic cells.

1360. chemotaxis

The act of a chemical stimuli to attract or repel; a process that causes some leukocytes to migrate to sites of injury.

1361. clonal selection theory

Explanation of how lymphocytes are sensitized to a certain antigen and how immune tolerance for self arises.

1362. clone

A group of genetically like cells derived from a single parent cell.

1363. cloning

Formation of a clone.

1364. complement

A group of plasma enzymes that catalyze a sequence of reactions against many different kinds of foreign matter.

1365. cytotoxic

Harmful to cells.

1366. DiGeorge syndrome

An immunodeficiency due to the absence of T lymphocytes.

1367. germinal center

Cell cluster in a lymph node that gives rise to lymphocytes.

1368. germinal epithelium

Epithelial cells that divide to form gamete-producing cells.

1369. graft

A tissue transplanted to a new site in the same organism or from one organism to another.

1370. graft-versus-host disease

An immune reaction of graft cells that destroys host cells.

1371. hapten

A small molecule that acts as an antigenic determinant when bound to a larger molecule.

1372. helper T cell

T lymphocyte that facilitates action of B lymphocytes in humoral immunity.

1373. hemolytic disease of the newborn

Antibodies from a previously sensitized Rh-negative mother destroying erythrocytes in an Rh-positive fetus.

1374. heterogeneity

Diversity.

1375. histamine

A derivative of the amino acid histidine released by injured cells that causes vasodilation and bronchial constriction.

1376. histocompatibility complex proteins

Proteins that give rise to antigenic individuality of a person's cells.

1377. host-versus-graft disease

An immune reaction in which host cells destroy graft cells.

1378. human leukocyte antigen (HLA)

One of a group of antigens that give cells a unique identity and that are used to match organ donors with recipients.

1379. humoral immunity

Resistance to disease produced by antibodies.

1380. hybridoma

A cell made by fusing parts of two cells.

1381. hypersensitivity

Abnormal reaction to a substance, as occurs in allergy and certain other immune reactions.

1382. hyposensitization

Reduction in sensitivity to a substance.

1383. IgA

An immunoglobulin in secretions.

1384. IgD

An immunoglobulin of unknown function.

1385. IgE

An immunoglobulin responsible for allergic responses.

1386. IgG

An immunoglobulin in blood and primarily responsible for resisting infection.

1387. IgM

A multiunit immunoglobulin most abundant early in an immune response.

1388. immune

Disease resistant.

1389. immune complex disorder

Hypersensitivity in which antigen-antibody complex damages tissues.

1390. immune response

Action of lymphocytes sensitized to a particular antigen.

1391. immunity

A state of disease resistance.

1392. immunization

Use of a vaccine or other procedure to create immunity.

1393. immunocompetence

Ability of the immune system to respond to a specific antigen.

1394. immunodeficiency

An absence or lack of a normal immune function.

1395. immunoglobulin

A protein that can bind with a foreign substance; antibody that binds with an antigen.

1396. immunology

The study of immunity and immune reactions.

1397. immunosuppression

A procedure used to lessen an immune response.

1398. immunotoxin

An antibody bound to a toxic drug.

1399. inflammation

Localized response to tissue injury, usually involving redness, swelling, increased temperature, and pain.

1400. interferon

A protein released by virally-infected cells that causes adjacent cells to make an antiviral protein.

1401. interleukin

A substance that facilitates or enhances an immune reaction.

1402. killer T cell

Lymphocyte that directly attacks cells with an antigen it recognizes.

1403. kinin

A substance that elicits events in the inflammatory process.

1404. leukocytosis-promoting (LP) factor

A substance that facilitates migration of leukocytes to a site of injury.

1405. lymphokine

A substance that stimulates activity of lymphocytes.

1406. macrophage

A large phagocytic cell in connective tissue.

1407. mast cell

A connective tissue cell that by releasing histamine initiates allergic reactions.

1408. memory cell

Cells that persist in the immune system after sensitization to recognize future encounters with same antigen.

1409. monoclonal antibody

An antibody to an antigen made by clone cells from a sensitized parent cell.

1410. naturally acquired active immunity

Immunity produced by having a disease.

1411. naturally acquired passive immunity

Immunity based on antibodies transferred across the placenta or in breast milk.

1412. passive immunity

Temporary disease resistance derived from antibodies from another organism (human or other).

1413. perforin

A cytotoxic protein that destroys cells by perforating membranes.

1414. plasma cell

An antibody-producing cell derived from a B lymphocyte.

1415. primary response

Initial response to an antigen in which sensitization and memory cell production occurs.

1416. properdin pathway

A sequence of reactions that activates complement.

1417. psychoneuroimmunology

A scientific field concerned with effects and interactions of psychological, neurological, and immunological factors.

1418. red pulp

The part of the spleen with numerous blood sinuses.

1419. secondary response

Rapid response to an antigen previously encountered.

1420. sensitization

Rendering a lymphocyte sensitive to a foreign substance.

1421. severe combined immunodeficiency disease

An absence of immunity due to a lack of both B and T lymphocytes.

1422. suppressor T cell

Lymphocyte that suppresses an immune response.

1423. systemic lupus erythematosus

An autoimmune response to a person's own nucleic acids, sometimes identified by a rash over the nose and cheeks.

1424. T cell

T lymphocyte.

1425. theory of immune surveillance

A possible way the body finds malignant cells and destroys them.

1426. transplant rejection

An immunologic reaction in which host antigens destroy transplanted tissues or organs.

1427. transplantation

Moving graft tissue to a new site or new host.

1428. white pulp

Lymphocyte aggregations in the spleen.

The Respiratory System

1429. Adam's apple

Thyroid cartilage of larynx, which is prominent in males.

1430. adenoid

Enlarged pharyngeal tonsil.

1431. alveolar

Of an alveolus.

1432. alveolus

One of many small air sacs in the lungs and in secretory parts of some glands; a tooth socket.

1433. anatomical dead space

Volume of respiratory passages where gas exchange does not occur.

1434. anoxia

Lack of oxygen.

1435. aortic body

Receptor in aortic arch that detects changes in blood gases and blood pH.

1436. apical

Located at the apex or tip of a structure.

1437. apneusis

Arrest of inspiration, usually to prevent overinflation of the lungs.

1438. apneustic

Of apneusis.

1439. arytenoid

Pitcher-shaped; a laryngeal cartilage.

1440. asthma

A disorder in which constriction of bronchioles causes difficulty in breathing.

1441. atelectasis

Collapse of lung alveoli or their failure to expand at birth.

1442. auditory tube

Passage that connect the middle ear with the pharynx.

1443. Boyle's law

Pressure exerted by a gas is inversely proportional to its volume.

1444. bronchial

Of a bronchus.

1445. bronchiole

Small passage in the lungs.

1446. bronchitis

Inflammation of bronchi.

1447. bronchus

An air passageway from the trachea to a lung.

1448. cardiopulmonary resuscitation (CPR)

A method for maintaining blood flow and gas exchange in a person with no heart beat and no breathing.

1449. Cheyne-Stokes breathing

Alternating episodes of rapid and slow breathing.

1450. chloride shift

Movement of chloride ions down an electrical gradient toward a region of positive charge.

1451. compliance

A structure's ability to conform to a certain shape.

1452. cricoid

Ringshaped.

1453. Dalton's law

Each gas in a mixture exerts a partial pressure that is independent of other gases.

1454. decompression sickness

A disorder due to nitrogen bubbles in tissues because of too rapid a decrease in pressure; the bends.

1455. elastic recoil

Return to original shape after being stretched.

1456. elasticity

The ability to stretch and return to original shape.

1457. emphysema

A disorder characterized by destruction or dilation of walls of alveoli.

1458. Eustachian tube

A passage that connects the middle ear and the pharynx.

1459. expiration

Exhaling; breathing out.

1460. expiratory reserve volume

Gas volume that can be exhaled after normal exhalation.

1461. glottis

A slitlike opening from the pharynx to the larynx.

1462. Henry's law

A gas dissolves in a liquid in proportion to its solubility and its partial pressure.

1463. Hering-Breuer reflex

A protective reflex elicited by stretching of lung tissue.

1464. hilum

A site on an organ where blood vessels and nerves enter and leave.

1465. hyaline membrane disease (HMD)

A lack of surfactant in newborns that allows alveoli to collapse.

1466. hypoxemia

Oxygen deficiency in the blood.

1467. hypoxia

Oxygen deficiency in cells.

1468. inspiration

Breathing in.

1469. inspiratory capacity

Total gas volume that can be inhaled.

1470. inspiratory reserve volume

Gas volume that can be forcibly inhaled after normal inhalation.

1471. interlobar

Between lobes.

1472. internal respiration

Gas exchange between blood and tissue fluid and between tissue fluid and cells.

1473. intra-alveolar

Within alveoli.

1474. intrapleural

Within the pleural cavity.

1475. intrathoracic

Within the thorax, or chest.

1476. laryngopharynx

Of the larynx and pharynx.

1477. laryngotracheal

Of the larynx and trachea.

1478. larynx

Voice box.

1479. law of LaPlace

Pressure that distends a hollow object equals the tension in the wall divided by the object's radius of curvature.

1480. lobule

A small lobe.

1481. minute respiratory volume

Gas volume moved into and out of the lungs per minute.

1482. mucociliary escalator

A mechanism in which cilia and mucus move debris toward the pharynx.

1483. narcosis

Profound unconsciousness induced by a drug.

1484. nares

Nostrils.

1485. nasal

Of the nose.

1486. nasopharynx

Of the nose and throat.

1487. oropharynx

Part of the pharynx adjacent to the mouth.

1488. palate

Flat plate-like roof of the mouth.

1489. partial pressure

Pressure exerted by one gas in a mixture of gases.

1490. perfluorocarbon

An oxygen-binding substance used in synthetic blood.

1491. perfusion

The flow of blood through vessels.

1492. pharyngeal

Of the pharynx.

1493. pharynx

Throat.

1494. phonation

Making vocal sounds.

1495. physiological dead space volume

Gas volume in respiratory passages not reaching gas exchange membranes.

1496. pleural

Of the lungs.

1497. pneumonia

Lung inflammation caused by infection or toxic substances.

1498. pneumotaxic area

A brain region involved in regulating breathing.

1499. pneumothorax

Infiltration of air into the thorax, which usually causes a lung to collapse.

1500. pressure

Stress caused by compression.

1501. pulmonary

Of the lungs or the blood vessels carrying blood to and from gas exchange membranes.

1502. pulmonary circuit

Blood vessel system that carries blood to and from the respiratory membranes.

1503. pulmonary edema

Accumulation of fluid in air sacs and other tissues of the lungs.

1504. pulmonary ventilation

Inspiration and expiration.

1505. residual volume

Gas volume remaining in the lungs after normal exhalation.

1506. respiration

The processes of ventilation (breathing) and gas exchange.

1507. respiratory

Of respiration.

1508. respiratory bronchiole

A small, thin-walled passage capable of gas exchange.

1509. respiratory center

A neural center in the brain stem that regulates respiration.

1510. respiratory distress syndrome

Labored breathing and impaired gas exchange because of surfactant deficiency.

1511. rhythmicity area

Neural center in the medulla that maintains resting level breathing.

1512. sinusitis

Inflammation of the sinuses.

1513. spirometry

Measurement of gas volumes entering or leaving the lungs.

1514. strangulation

Occlusion of a passage; choking.

1515. sudden infant death syndrome (SIDS)

Death of an apparently healthy infant suddenly and without known cause.

1516. surfactant

A phospholipid that reduces surface tension.

1517. tidal volume

Gas volume moving into and out of the lungs in normal resting breathing.

1518. tonsil

An aggregate of pharyngeal lymphatic tissue.

1519. trachea

Passage between the larynx and bronchi.

1520. tracheoesophageal fistula

A developmental defect in which an abnormal passage allows food to enter the trachea.

1521. ventilation

Movement of gases between the lungs and the environment.

1522. vital capacity

The largest gas volume that can be expired after a maximal inspiration.

1523. vocal

Of the voice.

The Digestive System

1524. absorption

Movement of substances across a membrane.

1525. accessory digestive organ

Organ or gland associated with and functioning with the digestive tract.

1526. adventitia

Outermost connective tissue layer on an organ or blood vessel.

1527. alimentary canal

Digestive tract.

1528. aminopeptidase

An enzyme that digests peptides from the amino end.

1529. anus

An opening through which wastes exit the digestive tract.

1530. appendicitis

Inflammation of the appendix.

1531. appendix

Worm-shaped sac at junction of small and large intestines.

1532. argentaffin cells

Stomach lining cells that secrete histamine and serotonin.

1533. bicuspid

Having two points or cusps.

1534. bile

Liver secretion that aids in digestion by emulsifying fats.

1535. bolus

A mass, usually a mass of food in the mouth.

1536. brown fat

Fat with a high energy content deposited around organs in newborn infants.

1537. Brunner's gland

A duodenal mucous gland.

1538. carboxypeptidase

A proteolytic enzyme that digests peptides from the carboxyl end.

1539. CCK (cholecystokinin-pancreozymin)

An enteric hormone that stimulates the gallbladder to release bile and the pancreas to secrete enzymes.

1540. cecum

Blind pouch.

1541. cementum

Material surrounding dentin in the root of a tooth.

1542. chenodeoxycholic acid

A bile acid.

1543. chief cell

A gastric gland cell that secretes pepsin into the stomach.

1544. cholecystectomy

Surgical gallbladder removal.

1545. cholic acid

A bile acid.

1546. chylomicron

A particle made of lipids and protein in the intestinal mucosa and released into lacteals.

1547. chyme

Semiliquid, partially digested food leaving the stomach.

1548. chymotrypsin

A proteolytic enzyme from the pancreas that hydrolyzes proteins into polypeptides and amino acids.

1549. chymotrypsinogen

Inactive chymotrypsin.

1550. cirrhosis

A liver disorder in which connective tissue replaces damaged liver cells; literally, orange.

1551. co-transport

Movement of two substances across a membrane by the same carrier.

1552. colipase

An enzyme that assists a lipase.

1553. colitis

Inflammation of the colon.

1554. colon

Large intestine from the cecum to the rectum.

1555. cuspid

A point or tapering projection.

1556. cystic fibrosis

An inherited disorder in which thick mucus blocks respiratory and pancreatic passageways.

1557. deciduous teeth

Nonpermanent teeth; 'baby teeth'.

1558. defecation

Passage of wastes from the rectum outside the body.

1559. deglutition

Swallowing.

1560. dentin

Bonelike subsurface substance of a tooth.

1561. diarrhea

Excessively frequent, fluid bowel movements.

1562. digestion

Breakdown of large molecules into smaller ones.

1563. dipeptidase

An enzyme that digests dipeptides to amino acids.

1564. dipeptide

A molecule of two amino acids held together by a peptide bond.

1565. diverticulum

Sac or pouch in the wall of a hollow organ.

1566. duodenal

Of the duodenum.

1567. duodenum

A short part of the small intestine adjacent to stomach that receives secretions from the liver and pancreas.

1568. emulsification

Process by which bile salts cause fat droplets from foods to break into smaller particles.

1569. enamel

Hard covering of a tooth seen above the gumline.

1570. enterogastric reflex

Neural signal elicited by excessively acidic or fatty chyme that slows stomach peristalsis.

1571. enterohepatic circulation

Return of bile salts to the liver and their resecretion in bile.

1572. enterokinase

A proteolytic enzyme from the intestinal mucosa.

1573. epiglottis

Elastic cartilage that closes the glottis.

1574. esophageal

Of the esophagus.

1575. esophagus

Muscular tube between the pharynx and stomach.

1576. falciform

Sickle-shaped; ligament that suspends the liver.

1577. fauces

Passage from the mouth to the pharynx.

1578. feces

Digestive waste expelled from the rectum through the anus.

1579. flexure

Turn or bend.

1580. frenulum

A small membranous fold that limits movement of an organ or part, such as the membrane under the tongue.

1581. fundus

Part of an organ farthest from its outlet.

1582. gallbladder

Sac on the underside of the liver where concentrated bile is stored.

1583. gallstone

Deposit of insoluble particles in gallbladder.

1584. gastric

Of the stomach.

1585. gastritis

Stomach inflammation.

1586. gastroesophageal

Of the stomach and esophagus.

1587. gastroileal

Of the stomach and ileum.

1588. gingiva

Gums.

1589. gliadin

A protein in wheat and some other grains that damages the intestinal mucosa in sensitive individuals.

1590. gluten

A protein containing gliadin found in wheat and some other grains.

1591. haustral churning

Motility that pushes the contents of the large intestine from one haustrum to the next.

1592. haustrum

One of many saclike regions in the large intestine.

1593. hepatic

Of the liver.

1594. hepatitis

Liver inflammation.

1595. hernia

Separation in a muscle layer; rupture.

1596. hiatal

Related to a gap or fissure.

1597. hydrochloric acid

Acid released from gastric mucosa and needed for protein digestion.

1598. ileocecal

Of the ileum and cecum.

1599. ileostomy

Surgical opening from the ileum outside the body.

1600. ileum

Lower part of the small intestine.

1601. imperforate anus

Retention of tissue that closes the embryonic anus after birth.

1602. incisor

A cutting tooth.

1603. ingestion

Intake of food or fluid.

1604. intestinal

Of the intestine.

1605. intrinsic factor

Substance secreted by the gastric mucosa required for the transport and absorption of vitamin B12.

1606. jejunum

Middle part of the small intestine.

1607. Kupffer cell

A phagocytic cell in the wall of a liver sinusoid.

1608. lactase

An enzyme that digests lactose.

1609. lacteal

Lymph vessel in a villus of the small intestine.

1610. lamina propria

Connective tissue beneath mucosal epithelium of the intestine.

1611. lingual

Of the tongue.

1612. lipase

An enzyme that breaks down lipids.

1613. maltase

Enzyme that digests maltose, a disaccharide from starch.

1614. mastication

Chewing.

1615. mesentery

A membrane made of two layers of peritoneum that suspends an abdominal organ.

1616. micelle

A small fat droplet in chyme.

1617. microvillus

A cytoplasmic projection of surface membrane of intestinal epithelial cells.

1618. molar

A large tooth specialized for grinding.

1619. motility

Ability to move.

1620. mucosa

Mucous membrane lining cavities and passageways.

1621. muscularis

A layer of muscle in an organ wall; the muscular part of the intestinal mucosa.

1622. myenteric

Of the muscle layer of the intestine.

1623. obstruction

Clogging or blocking.

1624. omentum

Two layers of mesentery located between certain abdominal organs.

1625. oral

Of the mouth.

1626. pancreas

A digestive gland that secretes enzymes and hormones.

1627. pancreatic

Of the pancreas.

1628. pancreatic juice

Fluid from pancreas containing bicarbonate and digestive enzymes for all types of food molecules.

1629. pancreatitis

Inflammation of the pancreas.

1630. parotid gland

A large salivary gland inferior to the ear.

1631. pepsin

An enzyme that starts breakdown of protein in the stomach.

1632. periodontal

Around a tooth.

1633. peristalsis

Wavelike, propelling contractions along tubular passageways.

1634. peritoneal

Of the peritoneum.

1635. peritoneum

A membrane that covers abdominal organs and lines the abdominal cavity.

1636. Peyer's patch

An elevated lymphoid tissue mass in the mucosa of the small intestine.

1637. pharyngoesophageal

Of the pharynx and esophagus.

1638. plica

Fold.

1639. plicae circularis

Transverse folding of the mucosa of the small intestine.

1640. portal triad

A set of three vessels (hepatic artery, portal vein, and bile duct) found in the liver.

1641. procarboxypeptidase

Inactive carboxypeptidase.

1642. pulp cavity

A chamber within a tooth that contains blood vessels and nerves.

1643. pyloric

Of the pylorus.

1644. pylorus

Stomach region attached to the small intestine.

1645. rectum

Terminal portion of the digestive tract between the colon and the anal canal.

1646. ribonuclease

Enzyme that digests RNA.

1647. ruga

Ridge or fold.

1648. salivary

Of saliva or glands that produce it.

1649. secretagogue

Substance that stimulates secretion of digestive juices.

1650. secretin

A hormone from the intestinal mucosa that stimulates secretion of bile and pancreatic fluid.

1651. segmentation

Splitting into segments; contraction of alternate intestinal segments.

1652. serosa

A membranous lining of body cavities that secretes a watery lubricant.

1653. sigmoid

Like the Greek letter sigma.

1654. sphincter

A ringlike muscle by which a natural orifice opens and closes.

1655. sprue

Inflammation and partial destruction of the gastrointestinal mucosa.

1656. stomodeum

Ectodermal evagination from which the mouth and adjacent pharynx form.

1657. sublingual

Beneath the tongue.

1658. submandibular

Beneath the mandible.

1659. submucosa

A layer beneath the intestinal mucosa.

1660. sucrase

An enzyme that digests sucrose.

1661. taenia coli

A lengthwise strip of muscle in the colon.

1662. taurine

An amino acid derivative that conjugates with bile acids.

1663. triad

Group of three.

1664. trypsin

A proteolytic enzyme from the pancreas that digests proteins into peptone.

1665. trypsinogen

Inactive trypsin.

1666. ulcer

Erosion of a mucous membrane, such as gastric or duodenal mucosa.

1667. ulcerative

Of an ulcer.

1668. unstirred water layer

Region near the intestinal mucosa where water molecules remain nearly stationary.

1669. uvula

Small bit of tissue hanging from the soft palate.

1670. vermiform

Wormshaped.

1671. villikinin

A mucosal hormone that causes villi to move.

1672. villus

Vascular tuft.

Metabolism & Metabolic Disorders

1673. amylase

An enzyme that digests starch.

1674. anabolic

Of anabolism.

1675. anabolism

Synthetic, energy using process.

1676. anorexia

Lack of appetite.

1677. beta oxidation

Metabolic pathway that oxidizes fatty acids.

1678. beta reduction

Metabolic pathway that synthesizes fatty acids.

1679. catabolic

Of catabolism.

1680. catabolism

Breakdown of molecules that makes energy available.

1681. cellular respiration

Metabolic processes that yield ATP.

1682. chemiosmotic theory

Explanation of how energy is captured in mitochondria.

1683. cholesteryl esterase

Enzyme that breaks ester bonds between a fatty acid and cholesterol.

1684. Cori cycle

Metabolic pathway in which lactic acid moves from muscles to the liver and glucose moves from the liver to muscles.

1685. deamination

Removal of an amino group.

1686. electron transport system

Enzymes and coenzymes in cristae of mitochondria that move electrons from substrates to oxygen.

1687. flavin adenine dinucleotide (FAD)

A coenzyme that carries hydrogen.

1688. gluconeogenesis

Metabolic pathway that makes glucose from noncarbohydrate substances.

1689. glucose sparing

Metabolism of fats by many cells that conserves glucose in blood for transport to cells that cannot metabolize fats.

1690. glycogenesis

Metabolic pathway for glycogen synthesis.

1691. glycogenolysis

Metabolic pathway for glycogen breakdown.

1692. glycolysis

Metabolic pathway for breakdown of glucose to pyruvic acid.

1693. gout

A joint inflammation due to uric acid accumulation.

1694. guanidine triphosphate (GTP)

An energy storage molecule.

1695. intermediate

A molecule produced within a metabolic pathway.

1696. ketone body

Acidic molecule that remains from incomplete metabolism of fatty acids.

1697. ketosis

Accumulation of ketone bodies in blood and urine.

1698. Krebs cycle

Metabolic pathway that oxidizes acetyl-CoA; citric acid cycle; tricarboxylic acid cycle.

1699. lipoprotein

A molecule made of lipid and protein.

1700. metabolic water

Water released from the oxidation of foodstuffs.

1701. metabolism

All chemical reactions in a living organism.

1702. nicotinamide adenine dinucleotide (NAD)

A coenzyme that transports hydrogen atoms or electrons in oxidation-reduction reactions.

1703. nitrogen balance

The situation in which the quantity of nitrogen entering the body equals the quantity of nitrogen leaving the body.

1704. oxidative phosphorylation

Capture of energy in ATP during oxidative metabolism.

1705. pentose phosphate pathway

Metabolic pathway that produces five-carbon sugars and reduced NADP.

1706. phosphorylation

Binding of a phosphate group to a molecule.

1707. respiratory quotient (RQ)

Ratio of carbon dioxide released to oxygen consumed.

1708. transamination

Transfer of an amino group from one molecule to another.

1709. turnover

Reuse of a substance made available by a catabolic reaction.

1710. urea cycle

Metabolic pathway that synthesizes urea.

1711. xanthine

A purine that inhibits cAMP breakdown.

Regulation of the Metabolic System

1712. absorptive

Concerning absorption.

1713. alcoholism

Disease of repetitive, excessive alcohol intake, which almost always leads to severe problems in daily living.

1714. anorexia nervosa

A serious neurological disorder in which a person loses weight and becomes emaciated.

1715. basal metabolic rate (BMR)

Rate of energy use that maintains body processes in an awake, resting individual.

1716. basal metabolism

The process of using energy from nutrients to maintain life in an awake, resting state.

1717. bulimia

Binge eating, usually followed by self-induced vomiting.

1718. calorie

Quantity of heat needed to raise the temperature of one gram water one degree Celsius.

1719. carbohydrate-craving obesity

Excessive body weight caused by a persistent desire for sugars and starches.

1720. core body temperature

Temperature deep within the body.

1721. diabetes mellitus

A disorder due to lack or inactivity of insulin that allows glucose to accumulate in the blood and urine.

1722. evaporation

Changing of a substance from liquid to gaseous form.

1723. frostbite

Tissue freezing.

1724. growth hormone-hypothalamic mechanism

A metabolic regulatory mechanism involving pituitary-related hormones.

1725. hyperglycemia

Abnormally high blood glucose concentration.

1726. hyperthermia

An abnormally high body temperature.

1727. hypoglycemia

Abnormally low blood glucose concentration.

1728. hypoglycemic

An agent that lowers the blood glucose concentration.

1729. hypothermia

An abnormally low body temperature.

1730. insulin shock

Unconsciousness due to an insulin overdose that suddenly lowers blood glucose.

1731. insulin-glucagon mechanism

A metabolic regulatory mechanism involving pancreatic hormones.

1732. kilocalorie

Heat required to raise the temperature of one kilogram of water one degree Celsius.

1733. metabolic rate

Rate at which nutrients are oxidized.

1734. polydipsia

Excessive fluid intake.

1735. polyphagia

Excessive eating.

1736. polyuria

Excessive urine production.

1737. postabsorptive

Related to metabolism after food from a meal is completely absorbed.

1738. pyrogen

A substance that causes body temperature to increase.

1739. satiety center

A neural center in the hypothalamus that regulates food intake.

1740. thermogenesis

Heat generation.

Nutrition

1741. ascorbic acid

Vitamin C.

1742. biotin

Vitamin required for fat synthesis.

1743. calciferol

Steroid having vitamin D activity.

1744. carotene

Yellow substance that usually has vitamin A activity.

1745. cyanocobalamin

Vitamin transported by intrinsic factor and required for normal cell division.

1746. essential amino acid

Amino acid required in the diet because the body cannot make it.

1747. essential fatty acid

Fatty acid required in the diet because the body cannot make it.

1748. folacin

Vitamin needed to help transfer single carbon groups.

1749. kwashiorkor

Malnutrition involving protein deficiency, usually in young children.

1750. malnutrition

Ill health caused by an inadequate diet.

1751. marasmus

Malnutrition to the degree of near-starvation.

1752. mineral

Inorganic substance.

1753. net protein utilization

Proportion of protein eaten that is actually used by cells.

1754. niacin

B vitamin used to synthesize the coenzyme NAD.

1755. nutrition

The act of providing substances needed for good health through food ingestion.

1756. obesity

Condition of having excessive body fat.

1757. pantothenic acid

B vitamin used to synthesize coenzyme A.

1758. pica

Craving for nonfood substances.

1759. riboflavin

Heat-labile B vitamin used to synthesize the coenzyme FAD.

1760. scurvy

A disease due to a vitamin C deficiency.

1761. selenosis

A disorder caused by toxic levels of selenium in the body.

1762. thiamine

A water-soluble B vitamin used to synthesize cocarboxylase.

1763. tocopheral

A substance having vitamin E activity.

1764. total parental nutrition (TPN)

Process of giving all required nutrients by a route other than the digestive tract.

1765. vitamin A

Vitamin needed to synthesize visual pigments and maintain epithelial cells.

1766. vitamin D

A vitamin that facilitates calcium absorption.

1767. vitamin E

Vitamin that acts as an antioxidant.

1768. vitamin K

Vitamin needed for synthesis of some blood clotting factors.

The Urinary System

1769. anuria

Without urine.

1770. arcuate

Arch-shaped.

1771. Bowman's capsule

Glomerular capsule of kidney.

1772. calculus

Hard mineral deposit, such as a kidney stone.

1773. calyx

Cup-shaped cavity or organ.

1774. clearance

Rate at which the kidneys can remove a substance from the blood.

1775. collecting duct

One of many ducts that receive filtrate from kidney tubules.

1776. cortical nephron

A functional unit of a kidney found mainly in the cortex.

1777. countercurrent mechanism

A process in which a system's outflow affects its inflow.

1778. cystic

Of a cyst or of the urinary bladder.

1779. cystitis

Inflammation of the urinary bladder.

1780. dialysis

Separation of molecules by allowing smaller ones to pass through a selectively permeable membrane.

1781. diuresis

Increase in urine volume.

1782. diuretic

Agent that causes diuresis.

1783. excretion

Elimination of a waste product.

1784. fenestrated

Having one or more openings; having windows.

1785. glomerular

Of a glomerulus.

1786. glomerular filtration rate (GFR)

Rate at which fluid moves from blood in a glomerulus to kidney filtrate.

1787. glomerulonephritis

Inflammation of glomeruli.

1788. glomerulus

A capillary tuft surrounded by a glomerular capsule.

1789. incontinence

Inability to control urine release from the urinary bladder.

1790. interlobular

Between lobules.

1791. juxtaglomerular

Of or near a glomerulus.

1792. juxtaglomerular apparatus

Cells near a glomerulus that help to regulate blood pressure by releasing the enzyme renin when pressure rises.

1793. juxtamedullary

Of or near the medulla, usually referring to the kidney.

1794. loop of Henle

U-shaped segment of a nephron where sodium chloride becomes concentrated in peritubular fluid.

1795. macula densa

Modified distal convoluted tubule cells associated with the juxtaglomerular apparatus.

1796. mesonephros

Temporary embryonic kidney.

1797. metanephros

Embryonic kidney that gives rise to adult functional kidney.

1798. micturition

Urination.

1799. nephrogenic

Arising from a kidney.

1800. nephron

Functional unit of a kidney.

1801. net filtration pressure

Pressure pushing materials out of a blood vessel.

1802. oliguria

Reduced urine volume.

1803. osmotic diuresis

Urine volume increase because of large numbers of osmotically active particles in the kidney filtrate.

1804. peritubular

Surrounding a tubule, as in the kidney.

1805. podocyte

Epithelial cell with footlike processes that extend around glomerular capillaries.

1806. pronephros

Most primitive embyronic kidney.

1807. pyelonephritis

Inflammation pelvis and adjacent parts of a kidney.

1808. renal

Of the kidney.

1809. renal clearance rate

Rate at which kidneys remove, or clear, a substance from the blood.

1810. renal failure

Inability of kidneys to remove wastes and adjust composition of plasma.

1811. renal glycosuria

Presence of glucose in the urine because of a tubule defect that prevents its return to the blood.

1812. renal hypertension

Elevated blood pressure because of renal artery constriction.

1813. renal threshold

Maximum concentration of a substance that can be returned to the blood from the kidney filtrate.

1814. renin

Kidney secretion that activates angiotensinogen to angiotensin I.

1815. renin-angiotensin mechanism

A mechanism that increases blood pressure and blood volume when either falls below normal.

1816. retroperitoneal

Behind the peritoneum.

1817. trigone

Triangle; a triangle in the urinary bladder wall formed by openings of the ureters and urethra.

1818. ultrafiltrate

Filtrate formed under high pressure.

1819. urea

Main nitrogenous waste in human urine.

1820. ureter

Tube through which urine flows from a kidney to the urinary bladder.

1821. ureteric

Of the ureter.

1822. urethra

Tube through which urine flows from the urinary bladder outside the body.

1823. urinary bladder

Distensible sac where urine is stored.

1824. vasa recta

Straight vessels, especially capillaries of the renal pyramids.

Fluid, pH, and Electrolyte Balance

1825. acid-base balance

Maintenance of body fluid pH withing a normal range.

1826. acidosis

Condition due to low blood pH.

1827. alkalosis

Condition due to high blood pH.

1828. carbonic anhydrase

Enzyme that catalyzes reaction in which carbon dioxide and water form carbonic anhydrase or its reverse.

1829. contraction alkalosis

Abnormal increase in the blood pH caused by a decrease in body fluid volume.

1830. dissociation constant (K)

Measure of the degree to which a compound ionizes into its components.

1831. electrolyte

Substance that ionizes and conducts electricity.

1832. fluid regulation

Maintenance of body fluid volumes within normal ranges.

1833. Henderson-Hasselbalch equation

Equation that relates pH to concentrations of an acid and its salt.

1834. insensible

Imperceptible.

1835. metabolic acidosis

Low blood pH due to a metabolic (nonrespiratory) disorder.

1836. metabolic alkalosis

High blood pH due to a metabolic (nonrespiratory) disorder.

1837. osmoreceptor

Receptor that senses changes in osmolarity.

1838. pK

Negative log of a dissociation constant.

1839. respiratory acidosis

Low blood pH due to a respiratory disorder.

1840. respiratory alkalosis

High blood pH due to a respiratory disorder.

1841. thirst

Desire for water or other fluid.

1842. thirst center

Hypothalamic nucleus that responds to changes in the blood osmotic pressure, causing drinking behavior.

1843. water balance

A state in which water intake and water output are equal.

The Reproductive System

1844. acrosome

Dense anterior part of a sperm that contains enzymes needed to penetrate an ovum.

1845. albicans

White.

1846. amenorrhea

Absence of menstruation.

1847. areola

Pigmented region around the nipple in a mammary gland.

1848. artificial insemination

Method for introducing sperm into the female reproductive tract without sexual intercourse.

1849. atresia

Absence of an opening; degeneration of oocytes.

1850. Bartholin's gland

Vulvovaginal gland.

1851. breech birth

Delivery of an infant buttocks first.

1852. bulbourethral gland

A male gland that releases secretions into semen.

1853. cervix

Neck; narrow end of the uterus adjacent to the vagina.

1854. chancre

Skin lesion, such as forms where spirochetes that cause syphilis enter the body.

1855. clitoris

Small erectile organ homologous to the penis located in the anterior vulva.

1856. colostrum

First fluid from a mammary gland after childbirth.

1857. condyloma

Genital wart.

1858. contraception

Prevention of conception.

1859. corona radiata

Radial arrangement of follicle cells around a mature ovum.

1860. corpus albicans

Scar that remains on an ovary after the corpus luteum degenerates; literally, white body.

1861. corpus luteum

Follicular cells that produce hormones after ovulation; literally, yellow body.

1862. cryptorchidism

Failure of the testes to descend from abdominal cavity into the scrotum.

1863. dysmenorrhea

Painful menstruation.

1864. eclampsia

Severe toxemia seen around delivery time, characterized by fluid and electrolyte imbalances and often convulsions.

1865. efferent ductule

A duct through which sperm move from the testis to the epididymis.

1866. ejaculation

Ejection of semen.

1867. ejaculatory

Related to ejaculation.

1868. embryo

Stage of human development from gastrula to eighth week.

1869. emission

Discharge, especially of semen.

1870. endometriosis

Disorder due to abnormally located endometrial tissue.

1871. endometrium

Epithelial and connective tissue that lines the uterus.

1872. epididymis

A coiled duct between efferent ductules and the ductus deferens.

1873. episiotomy

Surgical enlargement of the vulvar orifice to prevent tearing during childbirth.

1874. erection

Rigid state of the penis.

1875. estradiol

Primary human estrogen.

1876. estrogen

One of several active molecules that stimulate development of female organs and secondary sexual characteristics.

1877. Fallopian tube

Uterine tube.

1878. fallopian tube

Uterine tube.

1879. female pronucleus

Nucleus of an ovum that fuses with the nucleus of a sperm.

1880. fertilization

Union of sperm and egg nuclei.

1881. fertilized ovum

An ovum already penetrated by a sperm.

1882. fetus

Unborn child from two months development to birth.

1883. fimbria

Fringelike structure.

1884. follicle

Ovarian structure in which an ovum develops.

1885. fornix

Vaultlike space.

1886. gamete

Haploid cell; an ovum or sperm.

1887. gametogenesis

Production of gametes.

1888. genital herpes

A sexually transmitted viral infection that causes skin lesions.

1889. genital tubercle

A sexually undifferentiated protrusion that gives rise to certain parts of male or female external genitalia.

1890. genitalia

Genital, or sex, organs.

1891. gestation

Period from conception to birth (about 280 days in humans).

1892. glans

The cone-shaped tip of the penis or clitoris.

1893. gonad

An ovary or testis; organ that produces haploid cells.

1894. gonorrhea

A sexually transmitted disease caused by Neisseria gonorrhoeae.

1895. graafian follicle

An ovarian follicle.

1896. gubernaculum

A connective tissue band that guides movement, such as the descent of a testis.

1897. herpes

A kind of viral infection.

1898. homologous

Relating to parts of organs that correspond structurally but that may not correspond functionally.

1899. hymen

A delicate membrane over the vaginal opening.

1900. hyperemesis gravidarum

Excessive vomiting during pregnancy.

1901. implantation

Attachment of an embryo to the endometrium of the uterus.

1902. impotence

Inability to copulate; failure of a male to maintain an erection.

1903. infertility

Lack of ability to produce offspring.

1904. infundibulum

Funnel-shaped structure or passage.

1905. labium

Lip-shaped structure.

1906. lactation

Synthesis and secretion of milk.

1907. lactiferous

Making or conveying milk.

1908. lutein

A yellow pigment.

1909. luteum

Yellow.

1910. male pronucleus

Nucleus of a sperm that has penetrated an ovum.

1911. mammary gland

Gland that synthesizes and secretes milk.

1912. meiosis

Division of a nucleus that produces haploid cells.

1913. menarche

Onset of menstruation during puberty.

1914. menopause

Cessation of menstruation.

1915. menstrual cycle

Repetitive sequence of events involving ovulation and preparation of the uterus for implantation.

1916. menstruation

Periodic discharge of blood, tissue debris, and fluid from the uterus.

1917. mesovarium

A peritoneal fold that hold an ovary in place.

1918. miscarriage

Expulsion of a fetus before it is capable of independent life.

1919. mons pubis

Fatty area covered with pubic hair.

1920. myoepithelial

Related to epithelial cells that can contract.

1921. myometrium

Middle muscular layer of the uterus.

1922. oocyte

Cell that gives rise to an ovum.

1923. oogenesis

Process of producing an ovum.

1924. oogonia

Female germ cells.

1925. orgasm

An intense pleasurable culmination of sexual intercourse.

1926. ovarian

Of an ovary.

1927. ovarian cycle

Repetitive events of follicle development, ovulation, and formation of corpus luteum.

1928. ovary

A female gonad.

1929. oviduct

Uterine tube or Fallopian tube.

1930. ovulation

Sudden expulsion of an ovum from a follicle.

1931. ovum

Female gamete.

1932. Pap smear

A cell sample from the cervix examined microscopically to detect cervical cancer.

1933. parturition

Childbirth.

1934. penis

Male copulatory organ.

1935. perimetrium

Outer layer of the uterus.

1936. perineum

Region around external genitalia.

1937. placenta

Structure attached to the uterine wall that provides nutrients and removes wastes for a developing fetus.

1938. postovulatory

After ovulation.

1939. preeclampsia

Toxemia that can occur during pregnancy.

1940. premenstrual syndrome

Array of symptoms seen together a few days before the onset of menstruation.

1941. preovulatory

Before ovulation.

1942. prepuce

Foreskin of the penis.

1943. primary follicle

An early, immature stage of an ovarian follicle.

1944. primordial

Original or primitive.

1945. proliferative phase

A part of the menstrual cycle in which endometriual cells divide and increase in number.

1946. prostatic

Of the prostate gland.

1947. prostatitis

Inflammation of the prostate gland.

1948. rectouterine

Behind the uterus.

1949. reproduction

Process by which offspring arise.

1950. scrotum

A pouch in which the testes are located.

1951. secretory phase

A part of the menstrual cycle in which mucosal glands develop in the uterus.

1952. semen

A fluid containing sperm and secretions from the male reproductive glands.

1953. seminal vesicle

A convoluted saclike organ near the ductus deferens that adds secretions to semem.

1954. seminiferous tubule

A coiled tubule where sperm develop within a testis.

1955. Sertoli's cell

Cell type in seminiferous tubules that nourishes developing sperm.

1956. spermatic cord

A cord extending from the scrotum to the inguinal ligament that includes ductus deferens, blood vessels, and nerves.

1957. spermatid

An immature spermatozoan.

1958. spermatocyte

A cell from which sperm develop.

1959. spermatogenesis

The process of sperm formation.

1960. spermatogonium

Undifferentiated male germ cells from which sperm-producing cells arise.

1961. spermatozoan

Male gamete, sperm.

1962. spermiogenesis

Maturation of spermatids to become sperm.

1963. spontaneous abortion

Expulsion of a fetus from the uterus without external influence.

1964. sterility

Inability to produce offspring.

1965. stroma

Fibrous connective tissue framework that supports an organ.

1966. syphilis

A sexually transmitted disease caused by the spirochete Treponema pallidum.

1967. testis

A male gonad.

1968. tetrad

Four copies of the same chromosome temporarily attached to each other.

1969. theca

Sheath, such as that covering an ovarian follicle.

1970. ultrasound

High frequency sound waves sometimes used to create an image of a fetus.

1971. uterine

Of the uterus.

1972. uterine tube

A tube between an ovary and the uterus.

1973. uterosacral

Of or near the uterus and sacrum.

1974. uterus

A hollow, pearshaped organ where a fetus develops.

1975. vagina

Passageway from the uterus.

1976. vaginal

Of the vagina.

1977. vas

Duct or vessel.

1978. vas deferens

A duct between the epididymis and the ejaculatory duct; ductus deferens.

1979. vesicouterine

Of the bladder and uterus.

1980. vulva

Female external genital organs.

1981. yolk sac

Bag of stored nutrients in many embryos.

1982. zona pellucida

Translucent membrane around an oocyte in an ovarian follicle.

Genetics, Development, Life Stages

1983. adolescence

Period from the onset of puberty and adulthood.

1984. aging

Process of growing old.

1985. allantoic

Of the allantois.

1986. allantois

A fetal membrane that helps to form the umbilical cord.

1987. allele

One of two or more genes for a particular trait found at a given site on a chromosome.

1988. amniocentesis

Procedure for taking a sample of amniotic fluid from around a fetus to detect genetic or developmental defects.

1989. amnion

Membrane around a fetus that fills with fluid and acts as a shock absorber.

1990. amniotic

Of the amnion.

1991. autosomal

Concerning paired (nonsex) chromosomes and the genetic information they carry.

1992. blastocoele

Cavity in a blastula.

1993. chorion

Outermost fetal membrane, which is incorporated into the placenta.

1994. chorionic villi

Tufts of fetal blood vessels across which substances are exchanged with maternal blood.

1995. chorionic villus biopsy

Process of getting fetal tissue during development to look for genetic or developmental defects.

1996. chromosomal abnormality

Detrimental change in the DNA configuration in a chromosome.

1997. cleavage

Division into two equal parts; process by which a zygote develops into a multicellular ball.

1998. congenital

Present at birth.

1999. dizygotic

Arising from two separate zygotes.

2000. dominant

In genetics, a characteristic that appears in the phenotype whenever its allele is present in the genotype.

2001. embryonic disc

Trophoblast cells that give rise to the embryo.

2002. gastrulation

Development of three germ layers (ectoderm, mesoderm, and endoderm) in an embryo.

2003. gene

Functional unit of heredity; a site on a chromosome that transmits a particular hereditary characteristic.

2004. genetic engineering

Use of human-designed procedures to alter genetic information.

2005. genetic screening

Search for genetic defects in fetuses, newborns, and prospective parents.

2006. genetics

The study of heredity.

2007. genome

An organism's whole complement of DNA.

2008. genotype

Alleles of a single gene or all the genes carried by a particular individual.

2009. germ layers

First differentiated layers of embryonic cells; ectoderm, mesoderm, and endoderm.

2010. heterozygous

Having unlike alleles for a trait.

2011. homozygous

Having like alleles for a trait.

2012. Huntington's chorea

A dominant hereditary disorder that causes degeneration of the nervous system.

2013. infancy

The period of time from 1 month to 2 years of age.

2014. inner cell mass

Cells of a blastocyst from which an embryo develops.

2015. Klinefelter's syndrome

A condition due to the presence of XXY sex chromosomes.

2016. monozygotic

Arising from the same zygote.

2017. mutation

A change in genetic information.

2018. neonatal period

The period of time from birth to one month of age.

2019. neonate

A newborn infant.

2020. nondisjunction

Failure of replicated chromosomes to separate.

2021. phenotype

The appearance of an individual with respect to one or all inherited characteristics.

2022. phenylketonuria

A genetic defect in phenylalanine metabolism that causes mental retardation if untreated.

2023. point mutation

A change in a single base in a DNA molecule.

2024. recessive

In genetics, a characteristic seen in a phenotype only when genotype has only the recessive allele.

2025. reproductive engineering

Human-designed procedures used to alter the reproductive process.

2026. rubella

A viral infection commonly called German measles.

2027. senile

Suffering degenerative changes of old age.

2028. translocation

Transfer of part of a chromosome from its normal location to a location on another chromosome.

2029. trisomy

Condition of having three copies of a chromosome.

2030. trophoblast

Outer blastocyst layer that is connected with maternal tissue and gives rise to chorionic villi.

2031. Turner's syndrome

A condition due to having a single X chromosome (without another X or Y chromosome).

2032. Wharton's jelly

Soft, pulpy connective tissue of the umbilical cord matrix.

2033. zygote

Single cell resulting from a union of ovum and sperm; first cell of a new individual.

224

Index

For more information on other publications by Ed Creager, please visit the author's site...

www.edcreager.blogspot.com

and please note the author's "signature book" entitled,

"The Money-Saving Idea Book:
Inside Tips for Starving Students, Frugal Seniors and Every Financial Survivor"

www.ingramcontent.com/pod-product-compliance
Lightning Source LLC
Chambersburg PA
CBHW081112170526
45165CB00008B/2418